Communication
Skills for *Medical*
Professionals

Published by Walters and Worth, LLC
St. Petersburg, FL
www.waltersandworth.com

ISBN 10: 0615333966
ISBN 13: 9780615333960

Library of Congress Control Number 2010934159

This publication is designed to provide accurate and authoritative information as of the date of its publication in regard to the subject matter covered. Nothing in this publication should be construed as the rendering of health-related, medical or other professional services, or advice of any kind on specific facts. The information in this publication is not intended to create, and the transmission and receipt of it does not constitute, the formation of a doctor/patient or other professional relationship between the reader and author or publisher. You are strongly urged to consult a licensed health care provider or other appropriate professional, as applicable, for advice and assistance concerning your own situation or specific questions you may have.

Communication
Skills for *Medical*
Professionals

A CONCISE GUIDE TO SIMPLE, CLEAR
AND EFFECTIVE COMMUNICATION

MARK JEROME WALTERS, D.V.M.

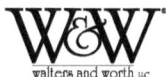

W&W
walters and worth llc

Contents

Nature has given man one tongue but two ears, that
we may hear twice as much as we speak.
——*Epictetus*

Introduction

A nurse tells a patient that a procedure carries "minimal risk." The patient sighs with relief and says, "So there's nothing to worry about."

"Not exactly what I meant," the nurse replies.

"But isn't that what you said?"

A dermatologist recommends taking a "very conservative" approach to a suspicious growth on a child's face. The child's mother is relieved. She didn't want the risk of a surgical scar. But the mother is taken aback when, in his very next sentence, the dermatologist suggests setting up an appointment for outpatient surgery.

"But you said we'd take a conservative approach," the mother replies.

"Exactly. That's why I want her in surgery as soon as possible."

Good communication is not always about what you say. It's also about what others hear.

In the first example above, the patient heard something very different from what the nurse said. The nurse said "minimal," but the patient heard "none."

This is not surprising. Verbal descriptions of risk are prone to misinterpretation. When you say "little" or "minimal," laypeople almost always hear "none." When you say "considerable" or "serious," laypeople almost always hear "inevitable."

In the second example, the listener also heard something different from what the speaker intended. "Conservative" is one of several commonly used words subject to dramatically different interpretations. To a surgeon, being "conservative" often means doing the most that is necessary; to a layperson, it usually means doing the least. To confuse the issue further, even professionals use "conservative" in opposite ways.

Good communicators also know that carrying on a conversation is more than simply taking turns speaking. It requires constantly monitoring a listener's feedback—verbal and nonverbal. It means being able to detect when listeners perceive a word differently from the way we mean it, and even modifying our own meaning in order to accommodate *their* meaning.

The communicators in the examples above fell short on both accounts—as many of us, in and out of the field of medicine, often do.

This book identifies many of the common miscues in exchanges between medical professionals and laypeople and uses these examples to highlight broader communication problems. The goal is to sensitize medical professionals such as you to communication issues and show how you can learn from your everyday experience with clients, patients, and laypeople. The aim of this book, then, is to get you into the habit of diagnosing and treating communication problems as naturally as you diagnose and treat clinical problems. Some would even argue that you can't practice truly good medicine without first practicing good communication.

Take jargon. Only by learning what constitutes jargon in the ears of lay audiences can professionals know when to use or avoid it. When it comes to paring down the use of such language, consider this book a diet plan for the linguistically overweight. But avoiding jargon doesn't mean communicating less. When a Mayo Clinic weight-loss expert was recently asked the one thing he'd tell overweight people, he didn't say, "Eat less." Instead, he said, "Eat more—more vegetables and fruits."

For those who may carry around too heavy a vocabulary for conversation with laypeople, this book frequently offers similarly counterintuitive advice: "Speak more, but use the right kinds of words and phrases," examples of which you will find in this book.

The book's recommendations are informed by two main sources. The first is personal experience. It was Yogi Berra who said, "You can observe a lot just by watching." As a medical scientist and professional journalist, I have observed a lot about finding clarity of expression within the halls of science and academia. This concise book—a sort of *Elements of Style* for health professionals—summarizes those findings.

I have also watched thousands of hours of video of medical professionals communicating (or not) with the public—and not just in medical settings but also in public presentations, media interviews, and other venues. I have observed a lot about how scientists engage lay audiences—or don't.

The second main source of the recommendations in this handbook is derived from the scholarly literature. Hundreds of studies of medical communication offer a lot of data, although, if one tried to summarize their conclusions in a small book, the work would generate far more contradiction and confusion than clarity. However, buried within this vast mound of research are scattered jewels of practical advice. I have tried to unearth and present them here.

In a few ways this book takes a novel approach to the subject compared to other books on medical communication. I have not segregated the medical interview from a discussion of ordinary conversation skills, as is typically done in other books. Although the patient interview has a special purpose, overstylizing this exchange has in some cases—in my opinion—done more harm than good, having led generations of students to view it as an interrogation rather than the conversation it is—or should be. Treating the interview outside the context of broader communication risks elevating it to almost a cult status, where the rules of simple, ordinary conversation might not seem to apply.

This book also differs from others in treating poor communication as more than just a sum of poor speaking habits—although it's those, too. Medical and other professionals often reap secondary gains from the way they talk. This isn't good for the patients and clients we serve, or, it turns out, even our own. Only by looking at those secondary incentives, I believe, can we hope to change our communication behavior effectively.

On the broadest scale, this guide comes down to a modern application of what Aristotle taught almost three thousand years ago: that people don't judge you just by what you know. They judge you by words that show you care—care enough to make sure they understand you and enough to make sure you understand them.

1

WHY COMMUNICATE WELL?

If you're a technically competent medical provider or a knowledgeable public health professional, does it matter much if you communicate well?

Study after study shows that it does, and in some surprising ways.

Patients widely believe that good communication skills are a key quality health providers should have, even though many believe that their own providers communicate poorly. (Beck, Daughtridge et al. 2002)

Medical ethicists agree but take the belief a step further: communicating well is an ethical obligation—no less so than giving patients good medical care. In fact, it's an integral part of good medical care.

Faulty written communication, often involving illegible handwriting, for example, kills many patients each year.

Acronyms or abbreviations can also pose risks. If someone tells a medical assistant to administer "MS" to a patient, and the assistant gives the patient magnesium sulfate instead of morphine sulfate, that's obviously a serious problem.

Beyond avoiding concrete medical errors that poor communication may cause, there are many other important reasons to learn to communicate as effectively as possible.

Trust is the foundation of relationships between professionals and their clients and patients. Technical competence alone, although it goes a long way, is insufficient to inspire trust.

Mutual understanding and affirmation are the essence of trust. We trust those who understand, believe, and value us. This is the ultimate subtext of every conversation. The exchange of facts or information is secondary.

In the age of digital information, as providers spend more time entering data with computer keyboards and less time conversing face-to-face, good conversation becomes more critical than ever. From a practical point of view, good communication plucks the most informational fruit in the shortest amount of time.

It is well documented that good communication also promotes healing.

The patients and clients of good communicators tend to feel understood, valued, and comforted. They therefore more readily follow medical advice than do those who don't trust the messenger. For example, those who come to feel they can trust the medical personnel they consult are more likely to change poor dietary or exercise habits, quit smoking, or follow other health-promoting recommendations. Consequently, they get healthier faster. (Beck, Daughtridge et al. 2002)

Good communication also promotes healing because patients and clients of good communicators feel comfortable asking for clarification if they don't understand something. Better-informed patients tend to heal more quickly than poorly informed ones.

Good communication has been associated with remarkable improvements in health. In one study, diabetic patients of good communicators had lower blood sugar levels, and hypertensive patients had lower blood pressures, than did the patients of poor communicators. Both groups benefited from a greater feeling of trust and emotional support. (Roter and Hall 2006) The way a provider communicates influences a variety of outcomes, including, in the words of one group of researchers, "satisfaction, trust, rapport, comprehension, compliance and adherence, and long-term health effects." (Beck, Daughtridge et al. 2002) Without trust, satisfaction and compliance suffer. (Roter and Hall 2006)

Clients and patients aren't the only beneficiaries of good communication. Health providers reap the rewards of having satisfied patients and end up themselves being more satisfied with their jobs.

Studies show that medical professionals tend to gauge success of communication by the information they collect or the speed or accuracy of the diagnosis. But patients tend to judge the encounter as much on whether they feel understood and valued as on whether doctors provide good care and treatment. Patients who feel understood tend to share more information, even if embarrassing. This gives providers more to work with, which itself also promotes healing.

There are also financial benefits of good communication. For one thing, it increases client satisfaction and reduces "doctor shopping." Good doctor-patient communication also lowers a provider's risk of being sued. Many medical claims ultimately stem from poor communication, including the failure to clearly answer questions. (Johnson and Johnson 2009) According to one study, poor communication, including failure to listen carefully to what patients were saying, was at the root of one-quarter of the malpractice suits examined. (Beck, Daughtridge et al. 2002)

Many suits stem from poor communication of risk in particular. You might intuitively try to protect yourself by avoiding statistics as much as possible and leaving wiggle room by saying something like, "In a very small number of cases, this or that complication may occur." But vague verbal descriptions of risk—phrases such as "may be," "perhaps," "not completely diagnostic," and "cannot be excluded"—leave the extent of the risk open for interpretation, increasing the chance of a lawsuit should something go wrong. (West 1984)

Surprisingly, the quality of medical care alone is not predictive of lawsuits. Poor rapport and communication are. (Moore, Adler et al. 2000) In one analysis, researchers consistently identified doctors who had never been sued and those who had been sued twice or more simply by analyzing their communication patterns. Sued doctors had shorter visits, interacted less with their patients to ensure understanding and ask patients' opinions, showed less interest in what patients had to say, engaged in less humor and laughter with their patients, and were less likely to tell patients what to expect from the visit. (Roter and Hall 2006)

Less than 2 percent of patients who have suffered significant injuries due to malpractice actually sue. (Roter and Hall 2006) Feeling unvalued, uncared for, and misunderstood is often what precipitates their seeking legal redress. As one study states, "It is the addition of insult, in the form of perceived uncaring or indifference, to injury that is often cited as the deciding factor." (Roter and Hall 2006)

The good news is that basic communication training can dramatically improve a clinician's communication skills. Studies show, for example, that decreasing interruptions and summarizing information are easily learned skills that can boost morale and compliance. Unfortunately, few providers avail themselves of these opportunities. (Rao, Anderson et al 2007.)

One study found that providers who had received basic communication training got higher ratings from patients on their communication style. Their patients more readily asked questions than did patients treated by doctors who had not gotten the communications training. (Rao, Anderson et al 2007.)

Why communicate well? Because it is integral to good medical care. And because your reputation, self-esteem, effectiveness, financial well-being—and even people's lives—depend upon it.

2

PRINCIPLES OF RAPPORT

The word "rapport" connotes harmonious accord, or a special connection or affinity between two people. Although often seen as the result of random interpersonal chemistry, rapport doesn't "just happen." It's created. And while not "by the numbers," its ingredients aren't mysterious, either. Somewhere between the mystery and the math lie its basic conversational ingredients. In other words, rapport can be created by almost anyone who learns the recipe.

Why, then, is rapport between medical professionals and laypeople sometimes hard to come by? Why do the parties often come together with the best of intentions, only to part with unsatisfactory results?

Professionals, many of whom dedicate their lives to helping others, rarely mean to alienate lay listeners. Our unwanted success at it is partly the result of the highly competitive process of becoming a doctor, nurse, veterinarian, or other specialist. In such an atmosphere, stressed and wary students learned to seize every real or illusory competitive edge. Language became the sword—and the shield. The professional etiquette that sought to conceal the weaponry merely drove it underground, to become subtly ingrained in the ways we learned to communicate professionally. Years afterward, it still spills into our conversations with clients, patients, and innocent bystanders.

Rapport depends upon a mutual sense of respect and even equality of a certain kind. No one is saying that the conversation between a medical professional and a layperson should be perfectly equal—or "symmetrical," in the language of linguists. That would be unrealistic in most cases. After all, people come to you as a medical professional because of your capacity to diagnose and treat.

In the vast majority of cases, you have superior technical knowledge. But you share equal standing when it comes to basic human dignity, or moral equality. And both you and your client or patient have—or should have—perfectly equal conversational rights.

Consider the graphic of the relationship between language, power and rapport on the following page:

Authoritarian

Patronizing

Stiff

Warm ———————————————— **Cold**

Warm and friendly

Distant

Solicitous

Egalitarian

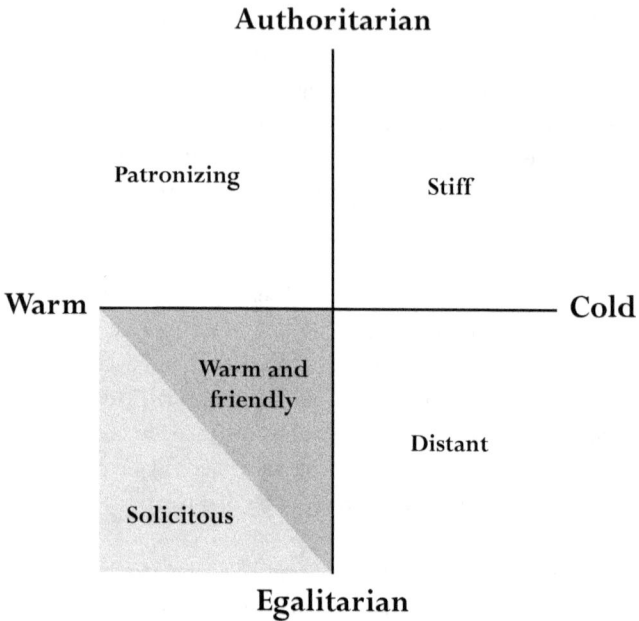

The above schema is one way to imagine the various ways that laypeople perceive professionals, at least as reflected in office encounters and conversations.

Laypeople may perceive the provider as a warmly speaking father or mother figure (upper left); they may see him or her as using cold, detached language (upper right); or their perception may be in between. While some may still find comfort in the traditional patronizing model of medicine, increasingly patients and clients see themselves as consumers buying a product—with the right to go elsewhere if dissatisfied. But paradoxically, their health is anything but a product, and so they don't want their bodies to be treated as one. Like all of us, they want language that reaffirms their humanity and intrinsic worth.

If we envision the ideal encounter as existing toward the warm side of the horizontal line and toward the egalitarian end of the vertical line, then we find rapport somewhere in the lower left quadrant.

Specific words and phrases can be used to help shape the perception of how you as a medical professional are perceived. Novelists, for example, have long known that if you want to make a character sound formal, you can eliminate contractions from that character's dialogue. If you want a character to sound warm and approachable, use plenty of contractions and put in a few colloquialisms besides.

By the same token, repeating the words and phrases that others use in conversation can help medical professionals come across as egalitarian, whereas sticking rigidly to our technical vocabulary (implicitly rejecting laypeople's terminology), even in ordinary conversation, can make us seem a little more authoritarian.

For a medical professional speaking to laypeople, the lower left quadrant may be the one to aspire to—warm and on the friendly side—but efforts to create artificial camaraderie are likely to backfire. Inappropriate language can make us come across as solicitous or diffident. Conversations in the lower left quadrant can be fostered by adhering to several principles.

1. Share "talking rights."

Conversational analysis shows that speakers use elaborate behaviors to claim "talking rights"—that is, to determine who speaks and when in the course of a conversation. Talking rights also include the power to introduce a new topic, as opposed to simply responding to one already on the table. In conversations with laypeople, professionals often claim a disproportionate share of these rights, which can sometimes lead to our dominating a conversation.

This includes, for example, controlling a conversation by asking question after question in expressions of "concern." Through this and other means, professionals in many different fields skillfully choreograph exchanges. We often lead the client or patient through the mazes of our own logic, expectations, and needs, all the while offering the illusion that we are there to hear what they have to say.

Although this is discussed in greater detail in the next chapter, you don't need a lot of details to know that to build rapport, you must ensure that all parties to a conversation feel that their talking rights are being honored.

2. Use verbal interruptions only as a last resort.

When the writer Robert Louis Stevenson eulogized his good friend James Walter Ferrier, he proclaimed him "the only man I ever knew who did not habitually interrupt." (Conklin 1912) If a trait is worth noting in our eulogy, it's probably worth cultivating during our lifetime. So rare are people who do not habitually interrupt that they are, indeed, memorable.

It would seem a no-brainer. We are told all our lives not to interrupt, yet we so often find it hard to resist. And this goes for almost everyone, not just medical professionals.

In one study, health providers interrupted, on average, within fifteen seconds after patients started to talk. They went on to interrupt 70 percent of the time. Interestingly, the patients who weren't interrupted spoke for only two and a half minutes on average. Interruptions, which are often used to push things along, did not shorten the conversations. They prolonged them. (Roter and Hall 2006)

Want to leave a good first (or subsequent) impression with clients and patients? Don't interrupt. But if you absolutely have to stop a rambler, use verbal interruption as a last resort. Try body language first. (See more about this in recommendation 42.)

Balanced conversations, in contrast to dominating ones, are marked by minimal interruptions, a more or less even taking of turns, and attempts to build upon what the other person says. Conducting a symmetrical conversation of this sort is like tossing a ball back and forth, rather than one person playing the conversational quarterback—as medical professionals often do, calling the plays and passing questions like a football.

Although egalitarian conversations can test the patience of harried providers, studies show that more symmetrical talk leads to more accurate diagnoses, more satisfied patients and better compliance. Balanced conversations build rapport, foster better relationships, and decrease the chance that your patient or client will go shopping for another provider. (Morris and Chenail 1995)

During a good-faith effort to get needed information, we simply may not realize we're dominating the conversation. This is where developing sensitivity to verbal and nonverbal feedback is essential. Just about everyone who feels verbally controlled sends out signals.

A person may become very quiet, raise an eyebrow or lean forward, hunch the shoulders or frown, open the mouth as if trying to talk, or raise a finger as if to press your "pause" button. (Morris and Chenail 1995) If you detect these or other signals, it's time to pause and rebalance the conversation.

3. Use simple words of Germanic origin rather than their complicated Latin-derived equivalents.

Want to be unintelligible to a layperson? Go out of your way to sound smart. If you want to sound intelligent, do what comes as counterintuitive to many scientific professionals: use simple, clear, concrete, and decisive language. The comprehensibility that comes from simple words radiates intelligence and engenders confidence in the lay listener. Big words often undermine both.

There is a reason why highly educated professionals tend to say, for example, "automobile accident" rather than "car crash." There are reasons why we say "elevate" instead of "raise" or "assess" rather than "figure out." It has to do with the history of language and a lot of social baggage that has tagged along with it. Words almost never convey just information. The words we choose can also be vehicles for conveying our social status. This isn't necessarily a bad thing; it's inherent in our culture and language. But overplaying the status dimension of words, often by using those with Latin roots, even unknowingly, can make us sound pretentious.

A lot of the more abstract words used in English are derived from Latin. In the Middle Ages, Latin was the language of nobility, the Catholic Church, and the educated. Latin was precise and abstract, qualities ideal for science, compared with the vernacular languages of the time. It signified high status. Latin also had shared meanings across time and national boundaries. It was about as international a language as there was at the time.

Words closely associated with Latin still form the vocabularies of academics and professionals in almost all technical fields.

The close association among Latin, social status, and the educated classes remains to this day. Consequently, professionals sometimes choose words to do double duty: getting information across while raising our status. Although most of the status lifting may be unconscious, it's not lost on listeners, especially if they speak differently.

How might the layperson's speech differ?

One of the interesting characteristics of English is that along with the Latin-derived words, we also inherited a vast Anglo-Saxon vocabulary, much of it derived from German, that was in common use among the uneducated classes of medieval Europe. Many Latin-derived words have a "low" German-derived equivalent. To this day, the Germanic words tend to be the simpler ones, with fewer syllables, and are more often used in everyday speech.

When a colleague at the office tells us something we already know, we might say, "I'm cognizant of that fact." But if a spouse tells us something we know, we're more likely to say something like "Yes, I know" or "Yes, I'm aware of that."

Here are some common Germanic words and their Latinate equivalents. A more extensive list is given in Chapter 4.

GERMANIC	LATINATE
ask	*inquire*
aware	*cognizant*
begin	*commence*
fix	*repair*
say	*articulate*

As educated folk, we tend to shun the Germanic words on the left side of the list, even though they often are clearer and simpler and sound more direct than our Latinate friends. Use of a lot of Latinate words tends to increase the social distance between us and our lay listeners; Germanic words tend to narrow the gap. Where we might unconsciously try to raise our status by "speaking Latin," we increase social distance at the same time. In a sense, distance is status in this respect. It's often an unproductive trade-off when it comes to good communication.

Listen to the difference between these pairs of sentences:

I wanted to inquire as to whether you commenced taking the new medication yet.

I wanted to ask whether you started the new medicine yet.

Please inform us if we can assist you.

Please let us know if we can help.

But there are occasions when the polite, abstract, and distancing nature of the Latinate is more appropriate than the gritty nuance of the Germanic. "Intercourse," for example, is always more appropriate in polite company than its Germanic equivalent. So are the words "urinate" and "defecate." But generally, replacing your Latinate vocabulary with Germanic words will make you far more approachable to laypeople.

4. Use some of your listener's words.

Aside from listening, probably the most time-tested way to build rapport is to borrow significant words and phrases from the speaker when you respond. This doesn't necessarily reach the level of mirroring what the person has said. But adopting just a few words from your listener can give confidence to a hesitant, nervous patient, or disarm a defensive one, and indicate that you understand what the patient is trying to say.

When they speak in English and you respond in Latin or Greek, you're telling them you don't speak their language. And if that's the case, you probably don't understand them very well, either. Make an effort to learn key terms in "their language."

If they say they're "afraid," then don't say "concerned." If they say "stomach," then don't say "abdomen." (Saying instead, "So where does your stomach hurt?" won't make you seem less professional or less educated. But it will show you to be compassionate and interested in the person's predicament.)

Using another's words does not mean trying to create false camaraderie by adopting the person's speaking style, replying to someone who says, "Ya know, man?" with "Yeah, I know, man!"

But insisting upon one's own technical or highly formal vocabulary during a conversation with someone who has a different conversational style risks coming across as upstaging, or even correcting, the listener. Borrowing words from the other can help build rapport.

You can also create rapport by using another's words to get insight into their way of thinking. Someone who uses phrases like, "Let me see if I understand" may be a visual thinker, while someone who says "What I hear you saying is…" may be more focused on auditory cues. Try to reinforce the listener's thinking style in words you choose.

5. Make your listener the subject of some of your sentences.

The most important word you can use in virtually every conversation with a client or patient is "you." There is no more powerful word than this unassuming pronoun. Yet medical providers often put themselves in the grammatical driver's seat (subject) and their patient or client in the back seat (direct object). Reversing the order (or dropping yourself from the sentence) puts the emphasis on the patient or client, and this can work subtle wonders on rapport.

DON'T SAY

I'd like you to lie down for me.

DO SAY

Could you lie down.

DON'T SAY

I know you must be wondering about the test results.

DO SAY

You must be wondering about the test results.

6. Don't confuse legitimate medical authority with superiority.

To be authoritative means to be recognized for expertise and wise judgment. To act superior is to believe you are better than other people. Authority is about knowledge; superiority is about power.

As a recognized expert, you should speak with confidence and authority. After all, there's a reason people place faith in your judgment—and that's what it often is, judgment—or professional opinion, as opposed to a black-and-white factual issue. But if the experiences of many patients and clients are any indication, it's easy for those rightful feelings of self-assured authority to be misconstrued as something decidedly less appealing: superiority. There seem to be certain junctures in conversations at highest risk for this misinterpretation.

Hints of superiority seem to arise most often when a speaker (1) tries to be emphatic, (2) calls attention to his or her learnedness, or (3) implicitly compares his or her knowledge with that of a layperson.

Speaking Emphatically

Not surprisingly, it is often when we speak emphatically that authority seemingly morphs into superiority. It's not surprising because that's also when we ourselves risk shifting from expressing an opinion to "knowing that we're right." It's one thing to forthrightly express an opinion. It's quite something else to convey, however subtly, indignation that someone would question our opinion.

Here are ordinary emphatic phrases:

In my opinion . . .
I believe that . . .
I feel strongly that . . .

Here are phrases that can be mistaken for superiority:

I can tell you that . . .
It's perfectly clear that . . .
There's no question that . . .

Calling Attention to One's Learnedness

The public puts a premium on cutting-edge medical knowledge and technology, and it's perfectly appropriate in some situations to let patients and clients know we're up to snuff. But overdoing it can sometimes come across as insecure (and insincere).

DON'T SAY
The latest information from peer-reviewed literature states that most people grow out of the allergy by their twenties.

DO SAY
Most people grow out of the allergy by their twenties.

Comparing Your Knowledge with a Layperson's
(See more on this at recommendation 18.)

We do it all the time—inadvertently.

DON'T SAY
There are lots of medical myths circulating out there. That's one of them.

DO SAY
A lot of people still believe that, but new information is challenging these beliefs.

7. Don't use code phrases for "Are we done yet?"

People tend to reply to canned questions with canned answers. Out of habit and with an eye toward thoroughness, providers often cap conversations with "Is there anything else?" or "Do you have any more questions?" Unless a client or patient is working his or her way down a laundry list of questions, you are not likely to get a meaningful answer.

In a medical setting, concluding a conversation with such a question can make you seem duty bound rather than truly caring or inspired. Nine out of ten times, patients and clients won't reply meaningfully and will be out of their chairs almost immediately. (West 1984)

If you have listened intently and the patient or client has fully aired his or her concerns, asking if there's anything else may be superfluous and misinterpreted as "Are we done yet?"

8. Be aware of "group talk."

One way providers, like people in other professions, strengthen their group identity is by using terms that continually reinforce it. It is the professional equivalent of "our family." But in reminding ourselves and our peers that we belong to an exclusive group, we also remind "outsiders" that they are not part of it. The vast majority of clients and patients are already keenly aware of this. It is part of the angst that people feel around medical and other professionals. Because they come as "outsiders" to begin with, emphasizing your own group identity, even unconsciously, doesn't do much for rapport.

DON'T SAY

As a physician, I know how effective antibiotics can be. But pediatricians like me are beginning to see how their overuse is beginning to threaten the public's health.

DO SAY

You and I both know how effective antibiotics can be. But now many people are beginning to see how their overuse can threaten our health.

DON'T SAY

Researchers have documented a number of unexpected side effects from this treatment.

DO SAY

People have experienced a range of side effects from this treatment.

DON'T SAY

Based upon the problems I've listed, I have some specific recommendations.

DO SAY

Let's work together to come up with some solutions to the problems we've identified.

9. Use inclusive tone and language.

As mentioned earlier, another aspect of power relates to the specialized vocabularies of various professions. Overuse of specialized terminology not only makes things incomprehensible; it also exerts control over the conversation. For example, by using overly specialized language and jargon, attorneys can unwittingly (or purposefully) discourage those not trained in law from participating in a discussion. Medical professionals sometimes limit access to—that is, control—a discussion in the same way.

DON'T SAY

There are a lot of options, and I don't want to give you too many choices.

DO SAY

Let's sort through the possibilities and see if we can figure out what's best for you.

DON'T SAY

The first lab result turned out to be a false negative.

DO SAY

The first lab result was wrong. It indicated a problem when there wasn't one.

10. Reflect, don't deflect, emotion.

Scientifically and technically minded people, who may be geniuses at dealing with information, sometimes start to drown when they encounter strong emotional currents in a conversation. Here's an example taken from an actual study.

Patient: *No, sir, I've never had a heart attack. Supposedly, I worked very hard when I was a young man, young boy. I was doing a man's labor, and I was always told I had a good strong heart and lungs. But the lungs couldn't withstand all the cigarettes . . .*

Physician: *Yeah.*

Patient: . . . *asbestos and pollution and secondhand smoke and all these other things, I guess.*

Physician: *Do you have glaucoma? (Morse, Edwardsen et al. 2008)*

And note the following exchange between the same patient and physician:

Patient: *Well, I'm not gonna have the operation.*

Physician: *You don't want to have an operation?*

Patient: *No. I can't.*

Physician: *Who told you that?*

Patient: *Nobody, but they told me if they open you up, if you've got cancer, once they open you up, you get poisoned.*

Physician: *That's nonsense.*

In each case, the provider deflected the patient's emotion—in the first case by changing the subject and asking an unrelated question, and in the second by dismissing the patient's fear.

It's on those points of emotion that the conversation should have turned—rather than ended.

3

LANGUAGE AND PROFESSIONAL POWER

Almost every communication—verbal or nonverbal—carries a scent of power, if for no other reason than that almost everything we do or say is meant to influence what another thinks or does.

In conversation, control usually manifests itself not as obvious domination but as using words and professional standing to subtly mastermind the outcome.

When it comes to conversations between medical providers and their patients and clients, control works both ways. To claim, as some observers have traditionally done, that it's all about the provider's power over the patient (or client) is naive and promotes stereotypes of patients and clients as passive, even incompetent, in the face of providers. (Ainsworth-Vaughn 1998)

Conversations often involve subtle negotiation. As such, they are often power struggles in miniature. Some of the negotiating "ploys" people—in and out of medical circles—use are obvious, such as interruptions (See recommendation 2) and the use of questions to steer the conversation. But one power-related technique in particular is well worth a separate discussion. This is the professional's use of "structural power" in conversations with laypeople. This issue extends well beyond medicine. It is present just about any time that professionals engage in conversation with clients.

Structural power comes from providers' membership in, or connection or affiliation with, institutions of power and prestige—in this case, the institutions or the establishment of medicine. This includes professional medical societies as well as socially legitimated "power," such as the right of certain providers to prescribe drugs. One could group this generally under the power of "medical license."

On one hand, such medical license is a powerful certification of competence, learning, and skill. On the other hand, at least as viewed by a lot of laypeople, the license can be exploited on occasion to unduly control conversation and, in some cases, to stake an implicit claim to general superiority. Although no responsible provider would make such a claim, some patients or clients might reasonably infer it from the nature of many conversations.

"Medical license" gives providers enormous structural power in conversations with laypeople. Unless you are aware that lay listeners may react to even subtle manifestations of this authority in your way of talking, it can make for misunderstandings, even hard feelings.

One of the ways structural power gets built seamlessly—almost invisibly—into conversation is through frequent, if unconscious, references to other providers, medical organizations, and myriad other reminders of the medical establishment. Among other things, this effectively keeps the conversational ball in the medical court and in turn plays to the strength of the provider and the vulnerability of the patient or client.

Take the actual case of Ms. Hazen, who came to her regular physician complaining of chest pain several weeks after surgery. (Ainsworth-Vaughn 1998) Referring to the surgeon, her physician, Dr. Miller, asked, "What does Dr. Marsh think that it is?" This was the first of many references to the medical "establishment" over the course of the ten-minute conversation.

There is nothing wrong, in and of itself, in referring to other providers and institutions during a conversation. They are part of the patient or client's medical history. But invoking professional affiliations can and often does serve the secondary function of building up the provider's authority while keeping the patient or client outside the established circle of confidence and credibility—even though, in this case, it was the patient's body experiencing the pain! This was not the one-to-one conversation it might have been. To the contrary, Ms. Hazen must have felt at times that she had entered a conversation with the medical establishment rather than with another human being.

But this didn't mean the patient was powerless. When Dr. Miller suggested surgery ("If they could go in and remove that..."), Ms. Hazen said, "I would be afraid to have him go in." Dr. Miller conceded, "Okay...I'm just asking."

Ms. Hazen then suggested hydrotherapy, but did so indirectly or perhaps by drawing on her own best source of power—her family. ("My kids were wondering if you thought I should be advised to have a whirlpool, hot tub.") Dr. Miller responded, "Oh... Take a deep breath in." He implicitly dismissed her idea and suggested she consider radiation.

It's worth noting during the conversation that Dr. Miller interrupted Ms. Hazen four times. She did not interrupt him at all. He also asked five of the eight questions during the ten minute exchange. And all of his questions were direct, phrased in such a way that an answer was required. ("Did you do anything exceptionally heavy?") He did not "mitigate" any of them, or phrase them in a way that would have given Ms. Hazen an out: "Do you recall lifting anything exceptionally heavy?"

Eventually, Ms. Hazen returned to her surgeon in an effort to figure out the pain. It turned out to have been caused by a pocket of fluid, which was easily drained.

It's only natural to speak from our professional vantage point, whether we are attorneys, engineers, or medical providers. That framework is, after all, a key part of our credibility. Throughout his conversation with Ms. Hazen, Dr. Miller reinforced his professional identity, perhaps unconsciously. Naturally, he sought to tap into various sources of his professional power, which were considerable. Given that laypeople sometimes feel on the losing end of conversations with their providers, how and when to use these sources of power is worth careful consideration.

Here are some recommendations.

11. When it's reasonable to do so, minimize the use of professional affiliations.

The influence of professional affiliations may be easier to see when we are faced with them outside our own professions. For example, imagine that you, as a medical provider who has not kept up on the financial markets, let alone retirement laws, consults a professional about your nest egg. Naturally, the adviser will probably structure the conversation around the constellation of institutions and professional affiliations that are most familiar to him and that ultimately serve his cause as an adviser. For example, the conversation is likely to be interlaced with references to IRAs, annuities, social security, pension and benefit plans, the names of insurance companies, various financial laws and the institutions enforcing them, recent changes in legislation, and more. He's granted the latitude, if not expected, to do this because he is, after all, a retirement specialist. That's the way many retirement specialists talk.

But this doesn't necessarily mean these references are required to meet your needs. In fact, the vast majority probably are not. Far from it: they shift conversational power to the financial adviser, who has fortified himself with these affiliations while discouraging your full participation in the conversation. The same principles may be at work when patients and clients come and talk to you.

DON'T SAY
Since the report came back from the radiologist today, I wanted to talk to you about his findings.

DO SAY
Let's talk about what the X-rays showed.

DON'T SAY
I can see from your chart that the surgeon at Hastings diagnosed it as scar tissue. It sounds like you disagree with that.

DO SAY
Dr. Marsh thought it might be scar tissue. What's your thought?

12. Use informal language when appropriate to warm up a conversation.

Although there's a thin line between talking casually and striking up false camaraderie, it may be a line worth walking. Informal language—even an occasional colloquialism—can quickly put a lay listener at ease and warm up conversation.

Informal language signals the listener: I'm relaxed. You can be, too. Formal and technical language can add fright to a routine condition or heighten the fear of a serious one. (Compare "gastroesophageal reflux disease" with "chronic heartburn.") (Young, Norman et al. 2008)

Some may argue that such informal language undermines professionalism and credibility. If anything, it can remind us not to take ourselves too seriously—something that patients and clients always appreciate.

Although the use of formal language is often simply a matter of habit stemming from years of formal education, it can also exert considerable power in a conversation even if unintentionally. The stylized syntax and vocabulary that members of various professions use is often emblematic of their fields. Among other things, it helps to heighten their exclusiveness, even helping to keep some outside the profession in a state of admiration, if not awe. Formal language can operate in a similar way.

DON'T SAY

I think not.

DO SAY

I don't think so.

DON'T SAY

One might wish to consider . . .

DO SAY

Have you ever thought about . . . ?

13. Use phrasing that invites dialogue rather than dampens the listener's willingness to ask questions or disagree with your assessment.

Depending on how they are used, certain words and phrases can have either a dark or light side. For example, "Of course" can signal to a listener that he or she already understands what you're about to say as in, "Of course, the next step is chemotherapy." But what if the listener is unlikely to understand what you are about to say, as in "Of course, we'll adjust the dosage based upon liver enzyme levels"? In the first example, the speaker serves the listener by acknowledging he or she already knows something. In the second, the speaker risks embarrassing the listener for not knowing something he or she "should" know.

The following are among these double-edged words, so be careful how you use them:

Obviously . . .
Of course . . .
As you already know . . .
I'm sure you'll understand . . .
It goes without saying . . .
It scarcely need be said . . .

Compare the impacts of the following statements upon a lay listener:

It goes without saying that you need a root canal on that molar.

You need a root canal on that molar.

The subtext of the first sentence is "Nobody who knows anything would dare question my assessment that you need a root canal." But the second sentence is simply a statement of apparent fact. Although declarative, it allows the patient room to respond without putting his or her ego at risk.

DON'T SAY
We should obviously increase the dosage of the medication at this point.

Were the listener to ask, "Why do you want to do that?" she or he would be put in the position of admitting ignorance about something the person should (at least according to the speaker) already know.

DO SAY

You should increase the dosage of the medicine at this point.

To say that something is "obvious" or "scarcely needs be said" likewise suggests that it need not be questioned or critically evaluated. When a dentist tells a patient, "It goes without saying that you need a night guard," the patient is far less likely to try to understand why. That may be one reason why medical professionals press the mute button so often. It minimizes follow-up questions, especially in potentially controversial subject areas.

The effect is much like that of a math teacher going through a blackboard of dizzying calculations only to announce at the end, with perfect seriousness, "The answer is obvious." The statement profoundly discourages any critical assessment of the teacher's work or even a call for further explanation.

DON'T SAY

It goes without saying that you'll need to be hospitalized.

DO SAY

You need to be hospitalized.

DON'T SAY

It's obvious that the fever is connected with the rash on his stomach.

DO SAY

The fever seems to be connected with the rash on his stomach.

DON'T SAY

It need scarcely be said that you should take this medication as directed.

DO SAY

It's important to take this medicine as directed.

14. Go easy on clubby or hypercorrect language.

Scientific professionals often use words and phrases that are almost universally grating to laypeople, in the same way that certain "lay phrases" grate on the scientifically minded. You can get away with them among peers. But to laypeople they can come across as snooty. While there is nothing technically wrong with the way you may say certain things (in some cases, you may be technically correct), they can needlessly stiffen a conversation and often distance the lay listener.

"Data are"

Technically it's correct to use "data" with a plural verb, as in "The data are inconclusive." ("Data" is the plural of "datum.")

But common usage persists with the singular: "The data is inconclusive." If you feel you must, stick to your hypercorrect guns and insist on using "data" as plural. But while you're at it, before you go to your next meeting, you might make sure you know what the agenda are. If someone says that the agenda is being sent by e-mail, make sure to point out that the "agenda are being sent by e-mail"—unless there's just one item on it, of course!

"High index of suspicion"

Scientists sometimes use this lulu in saying they suspect something. It's hard to find any logic in such pretension—other than an effort to give presumptive mathematical validity to an opinion.

DON'T SAY
We have a high index of suspicion when we see this kind of lesion.

DO SAY
This lesion looks suspicious.

"High degree of confidence"

Same tune, different words.

DON'T SAY
I have a high degree of confidence in this procedure.

DO SAY

I have a lot of confidence in this procedure. (If it's more than your opinion, then you might say so.)

"Admits"

In the language of medicine there is a peculiar use of "admits" in some contexts. When a provider, reading notes from a previous visit, tells a patient, "I see you admitted to frequent headaches in the past," the patient might sensibly reply, "Well, I never denied it in the first place."

15. Try to avoid problematic words with multiple definitions.

Ultimately, the meanings of words are determined by popular usage, not by a dictionary or language police. How people use a word determines its various meanings. In other words, dictionaries are more a reflection of the people's will than the other way around.

This is especially worth keeping in mind when it comes to a few problematic words that carry dramatically different meanings for scientists and laypeople, including your patients and clients. Even if they don't cause trouble outright, using them may lead to some confusion.

"Theory"

Most people trained in science understand a theory as a scientifically acceptable principle that explains a particular phenomenon. But to many others, "theory" may mean any idea thrown out there, as in "You got the theory that vaccines don't cause autism? Well, I got the theory that they do." Although it may be impractical to eradicate the word from your vocabulary in talking with patients or clients, use it judiciously.

"Conservative"

As mentioned earlier, when a surgeon speaks of taking a "conservative" approach to removing a potentially dangerous skin lesion on a patient's face, it means she will take wide margins in order to be safe. But the lay patient may think this means the surgeon will remove as little tissue as possible. To many people, "conservative" means leaving things more or less as they are.

Several years ago, when an epidemiologist from the Centers for Disease Control suggested that, "conservatively speaking," 3 million to 7 million people in the United States could die from pandemic influenza, he meant that would be the most who would be likely to die. But many people, including journalists, took it to mean that at least 7 million would die. To avoid ambiguity, the scientist should have said, "at most, 3 million to 7 million people would die."

Many scientists use "conservative" with just the opposite meaning intended here—all the more reason for caution about potential ambiguity.

"Fact"

The word seems harmless enough. But when scientists use the word, it tends to reinforce a layperson's misperception that a fact is an absolute, unchanging truth, because that's the tone in which they deliver it, even if they know that technically that's not true.

Unfortunately, the old saying that "a fact is a fact" is a myth. Facts evolve, depending upon the best available evidence. But many people don't see it that way. When a fact changes, or when one study disproves a previously held hypothesis, laypeople often believe that science is faulty and scientists are unreliable.

Scientists often compound the problem when they themselves present facts as if they were absolutes. They might say, "Here are the facts," when it would be better to say, "Here is the evidence."

"Uncertainty"

Although uncertainty is an essential element of science, to many lay people the word seems to have negative connotations. Therefore, rather than saying something like, "There is a basic level of uncertainty in scientific findings," it would be better to rephrase to indicate that scientists are open-minded, as in, "Scientists are open-minded, always ready to incorporate the latest scientific evidence into their thinking."

16. Respect your listener's level of medical knowledge.

Scientists usually blame communication breakdowns on lay-people and their general level of scientific and medical illiteracy. This blame game has a long and ignoble history. As the authors of an article in a medical journal in the 1960s put it, the problems arise from "such factors as the physical inability of the patient to hear what is said to him; his psychological unwillingness to receive unpleasant information or to impart information about private matters; anxieties and inhibitions stemming from perceived status differences or from uncertainties about the clinical situation; and his inability to remember clearly past experiences or to formulate and relate what he does remember," as well as "differences in ability to comprehend terms commonly used in medical discourse." (Samora, Saunders et al. 1961)

This contempt, sometimes manifested as condescension, seeps into the dialogue whenever we stoop too low to explain something—or don't bother to bend at all. Impatience with lay knowledge often comes out when we are questioned. As one scientist-observer wrote, "Scientists prefer to be treated deferentially, as experts, and not to be subject to that sort of probing. They—we—like to be regarded as infallible. We don't like confessing to uncertainty even when we know that we don't know for sure. And we don't like it when our claim to be disinterested is challenged. We don't like debating with our critics . . . who refuse to be overawed by men in white coats." (Rose 2003)

How can we break this destructive chain of mutual condescension and respect patients for what they do know, rather than making them feel bad for what they don't know? A few right words and a little humility go a long way.

DON'T SAY

Let me try to simplify this for you.

DO SAY

I may not be the best at explaining things, but let me give it a shot.

DON'T SAY

Pneumothorax is really complicated, and I'm going to try to explain it, but you may not understand.

DO SAY

There have been whole textbooks written about pneumothorax, but the bottom line is this: air in the chest cavity causes the lungs to collapse.

DON'T SAY

I get a hundred patients a week wanting antibiotics for the flu. Antibiotics are good only for secondary infections, not for flu. I could get into that, but it's probably more than you want to know.

DO SAY

It may be very confusing to people that physicians sometimes prescribe antibiotics and sometimes don't. In your case, you have a virus, and since antibiotics don't work against viruses, you shouldn't take them.

17. Beware of the wily "we."

Probably no two letters in the English language pack as much potential punch or convey as much nuance as "we." Depending on the context, the word can have opposite meanings. It can lift the morale of the listener or it can undermine it.

The "royal we" was once commonly used by royalty to refer to their own majesty. It still occasionally turns up in speech, even of nonroyalty: "We are a grandmother," British prime minister Margaret Thatcher said as she stood at 10 Downing Street. George Gale, a columnist for the Daily Express, responded the next day: "Watch it, Maggie. No one is indispensable, pride comes before a fall, some modesty and predence would now become you." (Lakoff 1990)

As it would become many of us.

"We" is an amazingly versatile little word. Depending on the tone and context, it can be inclusive or exclusive. The "inclusive we" means you and me, as in "Why don't we sit down and work out this problem together." The "exclusionary we" means me and my scientific colleagues but certainly not you.

When talking to lay audiences, scientists often use it in the second way, as in "We believe that patients will benefit from the new vaccine."

The "exclusionary we" can be a powerfully distancing word. It cools a conversation and sounds somewhat authoritarian to some listeners. It possesses the power and authority of numbers: "It's not just I alone who say this; it is all of us. So you'd better believe it." (Lakoff 1990)

The "inclusive we," on the other hand, is warm, inviting, friendly, and egalitarian, with the potential of uniting the speaker and hearer. The line between using "we" as an authority booster and using it when speaking or writing not as an individual but as a leader of a group or an institution is not always clear. But if your audience is not likely to know exactly who "we" refers to, it could come across as some invisible, somewhat mysterious, larger-than-life presence—that is, authoritarian.

Legend has it that the "royal we," or "authoritarian we," was first used in 1169 by English king Henry II as a way of saying "God and I." When experts use it, laypeople sometimes take it to mean pretty much the same thing. Pope John Paul II dropped the "royal we" from the English translations of his works and used "I" instead. You might consider doing the same.

How one uses "we" can clearly reflect power. After all, very few groups, mostly professional ones, have the power to use it at all. Imagine, for example, how you would feel if a patient said to you, "We tend not to agree with your assessment." When you say it, why shouldn't your patient or client feel the same way?

DON'T SAY

We think it critical that parents, educators, and health-care providers become aware of the choking game so they can look for warning signs.

DO SAY

My colleagues and I at CDC think it's critical for parents, educators, and health-care providers to know about the choking game so they can look for warning signs.

DON'T SAY

Unfortunately, right now we don't know how to prevent cerebral palsy. We certainly understand that those affected by this condition are anxious for answers.

DO SAY

Unfortunately, scientists don't at present know how to prevent cerebral palsy. Understandably, those affected by this condition are anxious for answers.

Yet another problematic use of this lowly pronoun is the "patronizing we"—sometimes known as the "infantilizing we," often used in talking to young children.

While many medical professionals may have embraced the consumer model of medicine, paternalism remains one of the most common relationships between patients and providers. (Roter and Hall 2006)

DON'T SAY

We'll have to put on a gown so we can take a look at your back.

DO SAY

Please put on a gown so I can get a look at your back.

DON'T SAY

Why don't we take your blood pressure now.

DO SAY

I'd like to take your blood pressure now.

18. Don't imply that a layperson's belief system is inferior to yours.

A common way that professionals unwittingly engender a sense of superiority—everyone does it at some point or another—is by measuring their beliefs against another's, especially a layperson's.

DON'T SAY

It's an old wives' tale that adults can't grow new brain cells. Science has shown that, in fact, they can.

DO SAY

Scientists once mistakenly believed that adults couldn't grow new brain cells. New research shows that they can.

DON'T SAY

From a statistical point of view, it's irrational to fear flying in a plane more than riding in a car.

DO SAY

Cars are so familiar that driving might seem safer than flying. But statistically, you're much safer in a plane.

19. Don't rhetorically tell your listeners what they must do, know, or understand.

"Lecturing" a person is a verbal manifestation of presumed superiority—or at least it can be interpreted thus, especially when professionals talk to laypeople. A sure way to turn a conversation into a lecture is to tell the other person what he or she "must" or "has to" know or do. Although they are rarely meant to come across as lecturing, try to avoid easily misinterpreted rhetorical flourishes such as "you must understand." This and similar phrases rarely add anything useful to the conversation.

DON'T SAY

People must understand that diabetes is a serious condition, with serious ramifications. It's important for patients, with or without diabetes, to take their health seriously and actively work at controlling their blood glucose and maintaining a healthy lifestyle.

DO SAY

Diabetes is serious, with serious ramifications. With or without diabetes, take your health seriously and work to control your blood glucose and live a healthy lifestyle.

DON'T SAY

One of the questions you must ask yourself is whether you fall into the category of unhealthy people I just described.

DO SAY

Do you fall into the category of unhealthy people I just described?

DON'T SAY

Parents need to know that the disease is still around.

DO SAY

The disease is still around.

DON'T SAY

You must consider the other factors.

DO SAY

There are other factors to consider.

20. Don't take evidence for truth.

Among peers, medical professionals usually express "truth" with extreme caution. They might say to a colleague, "The evidence weighs in favor of the procedure's effectiveness." They tend to be less cautious in expressing truth to laypeople. To a parent they might say, "The procedure has been shown to be effective." Both statements may be true, but the first is more nuanced. It draws a somewhat sharper line between truth and evidence.

Professionals probably are less cautious in talking about "truth" with laypeople because they are not as likely to get called on it. The problem is that it perpetuates black-and-white thinking among the lay public—either something is true or it's not, and we already know everything needed to decide the question. But science is about probability, not certainty. In casually talking about science as if it were black and white, medical professionals perpetuate the myth.

DON'T SAY

It's a fact that the hormone BST does not change the composition of milk, and you should have complete confidence in the milk supply.

DO SAY

All the available evidence indicates that BST does not change the composition of milk and the milk is safe to drink.

DON'T SAY

The drug is safe when used in accordance with directions.

DO SAY

Based on studies so far, the drug is safe when used according to directions.

21. Take note that a key reason lay people mistrust science is that studies sometimes seem to contradict one another.

This leads a lot of laypeople to think that science—medical and otherwise—contradicts itself with impunity. They have an excellent point—to an extent. A drug is okay one day only to be proven dangerous the next. A particular food or vitamin is shown to be healthy one day and then unhealthy the next. A beverage causes cancer one day, and it cures it the next. No wonder people are confused.

Scientists are partly responsible for this confusion because they have by and large failed to address what some people perceive as a double standard: apparently scientists are allowed to contradict themselves, but no one else is.

The broad generalization of studies in the media makes the scientist's work of communicating uncertainty that much more difficult. In many cases, the studies don't contradict but the generalizations do. And that can taint the science in the eyes of laypeople.

As a medical or other professional, you know that what some people perceive as a weakness of science—that it "changes its mind" all the time—is actually one of science's greatest strengths: its open-mindedness and willingness to respond to new data, even if it contradicts long-held beliefs.

When such a "contradictory" case presents itself—and contradictory studies are frequent when it comes to diets, medicines, and outcomes—we owe our listeners an explanation, if not for their sake, for the sake of science.

DON'T SAY

It used to be standard practice to treat almost all ear infections with antibiotics. That's no longer recommended.

DO SAY

It used to be standard practice to treat almost all ear infections with antibiotics, but that's no longer recommended. More studies have shown they aren't as effective as once thought—and their overuse make serious infections harder to treat.

4

JARGON

Jargon—highly specialized or profession-specific language—forms the core of much professional speech, especially in technical fields. Medical professionals, engineers, social scientists, attorneys, psychologists, and others all tend to use jargon. Not to mention car mechanics, computer technicians, golfers, and sports analysts. All of these specialists' jargon-based "dialects" are often indecipherable to nonspecialists in the field, sometimes even to people in comparable fields. The jargon of a biologist is likely to be foreign to a geologist, just as the jargon of a gymnast is likely to be Greek to a baseball aficionado.

To outsiders, jargon often comes across as gibberish and jabber. ("Gibberish" and its synonym "jabber," by one account, come from the name of an eighth-century Arab chemist, Jabir ibn Hayyan, also known as Geber, who allegedly penned more than two thousand books and treatises, apparently filled with—you guessed it.) (Shortland and Gregory 1991)

Jargon consists not only of words. Abbreviations and acronyms also make for jargon—sometimes dangerously so. Acronyms and abbreviations sometimes confound the very professionals who use them, especially in written communication. The abbreviation for "International Unit" (IU) is frequently mistaken for "IV" or the number 10.

So frequent are abbreviation and acronym errors that the Joint Commission on Accreditation of Healthcare Organizations has urged medical professionals to "initiate a campaign to eradicate the use of abbreviations in clinical practice" and "prohibit the use of abbreviation in all facility publications." (Brunetti, Santell et al. 2007)

Abbreviations aside, written and spoken jargon isn't all bad. By building on Latin and Greek roots, we can easily create extensive vocabularies and be understood by our colleagues. We know, for instance, that "ectomy," placed at the end of the name of an organ or body part, indicates its removal—as in "appendectomy," "tonsillectomy," and "lumpectomy." We need never to have heard the term "partial colectomy" to know what it means.

Socially, jargon also serves to strengthen group cohesion and identity. Jargon is a way of saying, "You and I speak the same language; that makes us part of the same brotherhood (or sisterhood) and different from the others." On the downside, language often strengthens cohesion within a group by pushing outsiders further away. And that can be a problem when we use jargon in conversation with a lay-person. What's more, jargon is often grossly overworked even for the purposes of internal communication, when professionals habitually choose the complex, sometimes pretentious word over the simple one.

As we have seen, jargon can push people away for the obvious reason that they don't understand you. But professionals also sometimes use jargon because it gives them control.

(Although jargon seems to get most of the blame for the breakdown in communication between laypeople and professionals, it's just one part of the problem. After all, if medical professionals stopped using jargon tomorrow, many of our communication problems would still remain.)

As noted earlier, one of the main motives for using jargon is rooted in the long history of the English language. If French belonged to high culture, Anglo-Saxon or Old English, with its Germanic roots, belonged to low culture. Even after the language of the French conquerors spread, Germanic words continued to be spoken by the English peasantry. But in time the French and Germanic merged. We often choose our words not simply to communicate but also to project status. In the medical professions, the Latin-based vocabularies predominate.

High diction may make us sound, at least to ourselves, more cultured and of higher status. Sadly, to the ears of most laypeople it can also make us sound a little pretentious or emotionally distant. What's good in scientific discourse can make for lousy personal conversation. Latinate words also tend to have multiple syllables, making them harder to say and understand than words with Anglo-Saxon roots.

Medical jargon can also make an illness sound a lot worse than it is. How might a patient react when a dentist says she needs to have an "occlusal adjustment" rather than to "have her bite adjusted"?

The upshot is that formal education shuns the inherited language of the peasantry, losing with it the social and communicative benefits of simple words with Anglo-Saxon or Germanic roots. They are not only shorter but also warmer, grittier, earthier, more direct, and more emotional than many Latin-derived words—just the qualities of good conversation that many professionals are sometimes identified as lacking.

The challenge for professionals is to relearn some of those ways of speaking in simpler terms that tended to be systematically eliminated during medical training. But surely, if we learned the Latin for common English words, we can retrain ourselves to use more Germanic equivalents in everyday speech.

You can usually tell the difference between Latinate and low Germanic diction if it's not already immediately clear. You can almost feel the difference.

How can you recognize jargon? Here are a few clues.

Jargon words often have a lot of syllables and they often take different forms, such as noun, verb, or adjective. (Germanic words usually play just one part in speech.)

Compare "converse" with "talk" or "demonstrate" with "show"—or, for a more extreme example, "walk" with "ambulate." (Well, not so extreme when you consider the common use of "ambulatory services," a shameless inflation that should simply be "walk-in services.")

Compare the following two sentences:

The automobile accident left the individual with multiple fractures, lacerations, and contusions.

The car crash left the boy with many broken bones, cuts, and bruises.

The first sentence reflects the speaking style of a highly educated professional. In the first, seven of the twelve words are polysyllabic, with a total of twenty-four syllables overall. In the second sentence, only three of the thirteen words have more than one syllable. There are a total of sixteen syllables. And various forms of the Latinate words, unlike most of the Germanic, often play several different parts in speech.

The abstraction of Latin-derived words also tends to make them void of sensory experience and hard to "hear" or "touch." For example, "crash" is a sensory word, while "accident" conveys more of a concept.

Finally, "boy" is personal, while "individual" is impersonal.

Here's an even more extreme example:

I conversed with my spouse and inhaled deeply prior to commencing my journey.

I talked to my wife and took a deep breath before starting my trip.

The second is more compelling because, among other things, it is easier to visualize and therefore to experience emotionally. The first comes across almost as a concept. The second feels more like a real-life event.

Latinate language infuses scientific talk. Here's a longer example of a highly Latinized (and wordy) passage pointed out in the Lancet:

Experiments are described which demonstrate that in normal individuals the lowest concentration in which sucrose can be detected by means of gustation differs from the lowest concentration in which sucrose (in the amount employed) has to be ingested in order to produce a demonstrable decrease in olfactory acuity and a noteworthy conversion of sensations interpreted as a desire for food into sensations interpreted as a satiety associated with ingestion of food.

Here's the Lancet's suggested rewrite:

Experiments are described which demonstrate that a normal person can taste sugar in water in quantities not strong enough to interfere with his sense of smell or take away his appetite. (Shortland and Gregory 1991)

(The editors could have taken the idea one step further by using "show" instead of "demonstrate" and "amounts" instead of "quantities.")

Jargon is so entrenched among professionals that any attempt to deal with it word by word would be like weeding the cornfields of Nebraska by hand. Words-to-avoid lists alone are futile. The best way to rid ourselves of jargon when speaking to members of the public is first to learn to recognize it. Once we can do that, finding a different word or phrase is often easy.

Most words you learned in medical school are jargon.

If there is a word you didn't know until medical school, consider it jargon. Although Latin heavily infuses anatomical terminology and forms the roots of numerous everyday words, three-quarters of medical terms derive from Greek, though many of these came to us through the more modern Latin. A number of purely Greek medical terms are still commonly used today: "hydrophobia," "nephritis," and "pleuritis," for example. (Banay 1948) But many others are best used to describe specifics of anatomy and physiology in scientific and professional communication rather than with the layperson.

Reacquainting ourselves with the most common Greek and Latin roots of jargon is probably the best way to begin improving our communication. By avoiding these roots where feasible in lay conversation, we can make a huge stride toward achieving clarity and rediscovering a common, Germanic-infused language.

Two broad categories in which medical terminology relies on Latin and Greek roots have to do with names of diseases, body parts, and medical procedures.

Names of Diseases

One important thing that distinguishes disease names from other classes of medical jargon is that many have become part of everyday language. Of the more than seven hundred Latin- and Greek-named diseases listed on the Centers for Disease Control and Prevention's website, many have become part of everyday speech. They have ceased to be jargon. (But even if laypeople are familiar with the name of a disease, it doesn't necessarily follow that they know what it means.)

Where necessary, consider explaining a disease by translating the Greek or Latin roots, using that as a launching pad for a more complete explanation. Aside from helping to define a disease, spending a little time with etymology can yield a treasure trove of engaging stories to spice up an otherwise matter-of-fact conversation.

"Appendicitis" means inflammation of the appendix. Your appendix is a small, worm-shaped outgrowth of your intestines. In fact, the word comes from the same root as the appendix of a book—something that's attached. The suffix "itis" means "inflammation." "Appendix" plus "itis" gives you "appendicitis."

The word "diabetes" comes from the Greek word for excessive urination. "Mellitus" comes from the Latin word meaning "honey-sweet." (Pepper 1949; Aronson 2005)

You could also point out that "influenza" comes from the same Latin word as "influence." Or that the word "ovary" comes from "ovarius," a slave in ancient Rome in charge of chickens and newly laid eggs.

A reliable and easily accessed source for the Latin and Greek roots of medical terms is the Online Etymology Dictionary at www.etymonline.com. Another source, if your institution subscribes to it, is the online version of the Oxford English Dictionary, at www.oed.com.

Names of Body Parts

In contrast to disease, most medical anatomy is based on Latin, thanks to the classic work De humani corporis fabrica (1543) by Andreas Vesalius. Unlike the situation with names of diseases, you can usually avoid anatomical jargon by using common names—once you become aware that you've been speaking in Latin.

Although you can't expect to simplify your speech by memorizing all jargon, you can familiarize yourself with a much shorter collection of the Latin and Greek roots on which much jargon is built. Learning to use the English translations of these roots where feasible can go a long way toward simplifying vocabulary.

The lists included here (abridged and modernized) come from a classic 1948 paper by George L. Banay, "An Introduction to Medical Terminology: 1. Greek and Latin Derivations." (Banay 1948) Simply reading them through, say, once a week for a month, will get you in the habit of identifying many of the most vexing Latin and Greek roots in everyday conversation.

GREEK		
Common Greek Medical Terms		
Root	**Common Term**	
aden	gland	
aorta	gorta	
bronchos	gullet	
cheir	hand	
chole	bile	
derma	skin	

gaster	belly
haima	blood
hepar	liver
hymen	membrane
kardia	heart
kephal	head
kranion	skull
larynx	voice box
mania	madness, frenzy
nausea	seasickness
neuron	nerve
ophthalmos	eye
osteon	bone
pepsis	digestion
pharma	drug
pharynx	throat
pleura	side, rib
pneuma	air, breath
psyche	soul
pyon	pus
Pyr	fire, fever
Sarx	flesh
soma	Body

spasmos	spasm
splen	spleen
stoma	mouth
stomachos	stomach
trachea	windpipe
trauma	wound

Common Greek Prefixes

Greek Root	Meaning	Examples
a-, an-	deficiency or weakness	apathy—lack of feeling; anemia—lack of blood
ana-, an-	up, upward, again	anaphylaxis
Anti-	against, opposed to	antipyretic
Apo-	off, away from	apophysis
Cata-	down, downward	catarrh
dia-	through, across, completely	dialysis
dys-	bad, difficult, defective	dyspnea
ec-, ex-	out, out of, outward	ectopic
en-, em-	in, within	embolism

hyper-	over, above, excessive	hyperemia
hypo-	under, below, insufficient	hypoglycemia
meta-	after, behind, change	metastasis
para-	near, alongside	paraplegia
peri-	about, around	pericardium
pro-	before, forward, in advance	prophylaxis

Common Greek Suffixes

Greek Root	Meaning	Examples
-ia, -iasis	pathological state or condition	mania, psoriasis
-ismos	condition	embolism
-itis	inflammation	otitis
-ize	treat with an instrument or drug	catheterize
-ma, -ema, -oma	concrete pathological condition	eczema, carcinoma, neuroma
-oid	form, appearance	thyroid—the shieldlike gland
-sis, -osis	production or increase	adiposis

Common Adjectival Greek Roots

Greek Root	Meaning	Examples
allo-	other	allograft
auto-	self	autoimmune
brady-	slow	bradycardia
caco-	bad	cachexia
crypto-	secret, hidden	cryptorchid
ecto-	outside	ectoplasm
erythro-	red	erythrocyte
hemi-	one-half	hemiplegic
hetero-	different, opposite	heterotonia
homeo-	similar	homeostasis
homo-	the same	homolateral
idio-	one's own, private	idiopathic
iso-	equal, like	isotonic
leuco-	white	leukocyte
macro-	large	macroglossia
mega-, megal-	great, large	megacolon
melan-	black	melanoma
meso-	middle	mesentery

micro-	small	microscope
mono-	single	mononuclear
neo-	recent, young	eoplasm
oligo-	little, few	oligopnea
ortho-	straight, correct	orthopedics
oxy-	sharp, acid	oxylalia
pan-	all, entire	pancreas
polio-	gray	polioencephalitis
poly-	much, many	polyuria
proto-	first	prototype
pseudo-	false	pseudocyesis
tachy-	fast	tachycardia
xantho-	yellow	xanthoderm

Common Adverbial Greek Roots		
Greek Root	Meaning	Examples
di-	twice	dimorphism
endo-	within	endometrium
eu-	well, easy	euphoric
exo-	outside, outward	exogenous
opisth-	behind	opisthotonos
palin-	backward, again	palinesthesia
tele-	distant	teleneuron

Greek Roots as Parts of Compound Words

Greek Root	Meaning	Examples
-agra	seizure	cardiagra
-algia	pain	neuralgia
-asthenia	weakness	myasthenia
-cele	protrusion, tumor, hernia	hydrocele
-cinesia	movement	enterocinesia
-clasia	breaking	hemoclasis
-cyte	cell	erythrocyte
-ectomy	excision	hysterectomy
-emia	blood	anemia
-esthesia	feeling, sensibility	paresthesia
-genesis	generation	spermatogenesis
-gram	drawing	cardiogram
-graph	write	ventriculograph
-lith	stone, calculus	enterolith
-logia	discourse, treatise	urology
-lysis	breaking down	hemolysis
-malacia	softening	osteomalacia
-mania	madness	kleptomania

-megalia	large	splenomegaly
-meter	instrument for measuring	Thermometer
-odynia	pain	otodynia
-opia	vision	myopia
-pathy	suffering	adenopathy
-philia	to like	hemophilia
-phobia	fear	claustrophobia
-plasty	to form	rhinoplasty
-plegia	stroke	hemiplegia
-poiesis	formation	hematopoiesis
-ptosis	displacement	hysteroptosis
-pyosis	pus	arthropyosis
-rrhagia, -rrhage	to break forth	hemorrhage
-rrhaphy	stitch	perineorrhaphy
-rrhea	flow	gonorrhea
-sclerosis	hardening	arteriosclerosis
-scope, -scopy	to view	ophthalmoscope
-spasm	cramp	pylorospasm
-stasis	stoppage	hemostasis
-staxis	dripping	epistaxis
-stenosis	narrowing	enterostenosis

-stomy	mouth	colostomy
-therapy	treatment	hydrotherapy
-thermy	heat	diathermy
-tomy	incision	laparotomy
-trophy	to nourish	hypertrophy
-uria	urinate	hematuria

LATIN

Common Latin Word Roots

Latin Root	Common Term	
anus	ring	
aqua	water	
bacillus	little rod	
bucca	cheek	
caput	head	
caries	decay	
cella	chamber	
cerebrum	brain	
cervix	neck	
cor	heart	
corpus	body	
cortex	bark	
cutis	skin	

dens	tooth
facies	face
fascia	band
febris	fever
femur	thigh
foramen	perforation
fornix	arch
fossa	ditch
frons	forehead
fundus	base, bottom
glans	gland
hernia	rupture
ilium	flank
labium	lip
latus	side
lens	lentil
ligamentum	binding
lingua	tongue
lues	plague
lupus	wolf
manus	hand
meatus	opening
mens	mind

mensis	month
morbus	disease
nodus	knot
oculus	eye
os	mouth
ovum	egg
patella	shallow pan
pectus	chest
pelvis	basin
placenta	flat cake
pons	bridge
pulmo	lung
pupilla	little girl
ren	kidney
retina	net
ruga	wrinkle, furrow
saliva	spittle
scrotum	pouch
sella	chair
semen	seed
spina	thorn
stimulus	goad
succus	juice

sudor	sweat
tabes	wasting
talus	ankle
tergum	back
tonsilla	pointed pole
tunica	garment
tussis	cough
ulcus	ulcer
uterus	womb
vagina	sheath
valva	valve
vas	vessel
vena	vein
venter	belly
vermis	worm
vesica	bladder
virus	poison

Common Latin Prefixes

Latin Root	Meaning
a-, ab-, abs-	away from, off
ad-	to, toward
ambi-, ambo-	both, on both sides
ante-	before, in front of, forward
bi-, bis-	twice, double
circum-	around, about
co-, con-	with, together
contra-	against, opposed
de-	down, downward
e-, ec-, ex-	out, out of, off, removal
in-, im-	in, into, inside
infra-	below, beneath, downward, lower
inter-	between
intra-	within, inside
intro-	into, inward, within
juxta-	beside, near

ob-	in front of, against, near (in space or time)
per-	through, thorough, excessive
prae-, pre-	before, in front of
pro-	before, in front of, forward
re-, red-	back, again
retro-	back, backward, behind
sub-, sup-	beneath, downward, nearly
super-	above (in position or degree)
supra-	above, upon, over, upper
trans-	across, through, beyond
ultra-	beyond, in excess

Common Latin Adjectives

Latin Root	Meaning	
albo-	white	
anter-	before, in front of	
dextro-	right	
mal-	bad, evil	
medio-	middle	
multi-	many	
pluri-	more	
postero-	behind	
primi-	first	
semi-	half, in part	
sesqui-	one and a half, one-half more	
sinistro-	left	
uni-	one	

5

ART OF THE EXPLANATION

Health professionals are trained to understand difficult concepts, not explain them to others—or at least not to nonscientists. The best way to minimize the need for long explanations is to use simple words in the first place. Big words beget big explanations. But sometimes you will need to use a big word. When you do, get in the habit of explaining it on the spot, with a simple clause, if possible.

DON'T SAY

In vitro, the medication prevents immune cells from releasing histamines. It doesn't work in vivo.

DO SAY

In test tubes, the medicine prevents immune cells from releasing histamines—chemicals that cause allergic reactions. There's no evidence that it works in humans.

In the second example, the problematic "in vitro" is replaced with the easily understood "in test tubes." "Histamines" is retained but explained as "chemicals that cause allergic reactions." If that preemptive clause were omitted, the listener would probably ask, "What's a histamine?" And then, with the question hanging in the air, you would be apt—if not obligated—to give a much longer explanation. If you get in the habit of avoiding big words where you can and explaining required ones then and there with a single clause, you can greatly reduce the need to get into detailed explanations in the first place.

In some cases, eliminating big words and giving clear definitions won't avert the need for longer explanations. If a patient is about to undergo an unfamiliar procedure, you'll probably need to explain things.

You can't memorize or otherwise prepare yourself for every explanation you'll have to give, but it's a good idea to make a list of the most common ones you encounter. Then it's sometimes helpful to follow a standardized approach in explaining things. Should a new challenge arise, at least you'll have a familiar process in mind.

22. Try the three-stage explanation technique.

Many of the most lucid explanations neatly unfold in three stages, telling what something is, what it does, and then how it works. Each stage may need only one sentence to convey the essence.

Here's a classic three-stage explanation from the Centers for Disease Control and Prevention's website:

Epilepsy is a chronic neurological condition characterized by recurrent seizures. (What it is.)

There are many types of seizures and their symptoms can vary from a momentary disruption of the senses, to short periods of unconsciousness or staring spells, to convulsions. (What it does.)

Epilepsy can be caused by many different conditions that affect a person's brain. Often no definite cause can be found. (How it does it.)

Just as diseases often lend themselves to neat three-stage explanations, so do medical procedures. Here's one from the Mayo Clinic:

Coronary angioplasty . . . is a procedure (what it is) used to open clogged heart arteries (what it does). Angioplasty involves temporarily inserting and blowing up a tiny balloon where your artery is clogged to help widen the artery (How it does it).

For practice, here are some more examples broken down into the stages:

Stage 1. Tell what something is.
A catheter is a small, flexible tube that can be inserted into a body cavity, duct, or vessel.

Stage 2. Tell what something does.
It allows fluids to drain out or is used to make a passageway bigger.

Stage 3. Tell how it does it.
A catheter drains fluids by providing a clear passageway. It can expand a passageway as it's pushed through and keep it open while the fluid drains out.

Here's a three-stage explanation of a complete blood count (CBC).

1. What it is: *A CBC, or complete blood count, is a routine test of the various cells in your blood, especially the white cells and the red blood cells.*

2. What it does: *The CBC measures the numbers of these cells and determines if they are normal or abnormal.*

3. How it does it: *In a CBC, the blood cells are counted, measured and analyzed by a machine, which then prints out a report.*

Finally, here's a three-stage explanation of an endoscope:

1. What it is: *An endoscope is a flexible tube with an eyepiece at one end and a miniature light and lens at the other.*

2. What it does: *It lets us look into the body without the need for surgery.*

3. How it does it: *The endoscope is inserted into a body opening, such as the mouth or rectum, and then gently pushed into the canal to see if it's normal or not.*

Mixing up the various stages of an explanation—telling someone a little about what it does and how it works, and then a bit more about what it is—may foster confusion. Logically, someone needs to visualize something before they can conceptualize what it does and how it works.

Here's an example of a mangled CBC explanation:

The CBC measures the numbers of these cells and determines if they are normal or abnormal. A machine prints out a report. The blood cells are counted and measured and chemically analyzed. It's a routine test of the various cells in your blood, especially the white cells and the red blood cells.

Here's an example of a mangled endoscope explanation:

An endoscope lets us look into the body without the need for surgery. The endoscope is inserted into a body opening, such as the mouth or rectum. It's a flexible tube with an eyepiece at one end and a miniature light and lens at the other that is gently pushed into the canal so we can look at it to see if it's normal or not.

23. Use analogies to bolster your explanations.

One of the most powerful ways to strengthen an explanation is to use analogies.

Evidence suggests that appropriate analogies, or comparisons, help science students learn scientific material more quickly and with better conceptual understanding. (Frieden and Dolev 2005) In some instances, analogies also convey emotion—fear, joy, desperation, hope—and can thereby become the ultimate multichannel communication device.

Telling a child that her newly diagnosed leukemia is like a weed in a flower garden conveys information—and emotion—at many levels. Explaining that her doctors are like gardeners is a way of assuring her not only that she is beautiful (like a garden) but also that she will be well cared for. Compare this with likening leukemia to, for example, a bully in the classroom.

An analogy draws its power from recasting something unfamiliar into something commonplace. Many of our understandings of science are built on analogies. Using a zipper to explain the separating of DNA's double helix is one of the most famous analogies in science, as is the twisted ladder explaining DNA's three-dimensional structure. Other well-known scientific analogies include comparing mitochondria to a powerhouse, the heart and circulatory system to the plumbing in a house, and sound waves to ripples on a pond.

Charles Darwin often used comparisons. In The Origin of Species he compared evolutionary lineages to branches of a tree:

The green and budding twigs may represent existing species; and those produced during each former year may represent the long succession of extinct species. As buds give rise by growth to fresh buds, and these, if vigorous, branch out and overtop on all a feebler branch, so by generation I believe it has been with the Tree of Life.

Although the tone may seem dated (it was published in 1859), the point remains. Analogies not only simplify concepts but also can make them memorable.

Health and medicine have produced a wealth of analogies, but perhaps no field has contributed more than dermatology. Consider the following excerpts from an article in the Journal of the American Academy of Dermatology (Frieden and Dolev 2005), followed by my critiques.

Venous and capillary malformations: *like a faulty plumbing system. Over time, the backup can slowly get worse and the problem can progress.*

This makes the point effectively.

Granuloma annulare: *Like teenagers at a convenience store on a Saturday night, the white blood cells are gathered in the middle layer of the skin and cause trouble, just because they are there.*

This is a poor analogy because it doesn't explain anything about why the white blood cells congregate. Furthermore, to villainize teenagers for hanging out serves no relevant purpose.

Hemangioma: *Like a Polaroid photograph, hemangiomas are invisible at birth and need time to become fully apparent.*

Although an apt analogy at one time, likening something to a developing Polaroid photograph may be of limited value to those who have grown up in the digital age of instant images.

Analogies can be a great boost to understanding, but only if they are truly apt. Compare the two below.

Taking medicines: *Taking your prescription is like watering a garden. If you wait until the plants have wilted, it's too late. Water every day.*

This unfortunate analogy suggests we need medicine as regularly as plants need water, although it would probably be okay if the patient is on a daily regimen for life.

Aneurism: *An aneurism is like an inner tube inside a tire. If the tire is cut, the inner tube bulges. This weak spot in the tire could blow at any time.*

This is a good analogy that captures the mechanics of an aneurism while conveying its risks—albeit in a dramatic way.

24. Use word derivations to boost your explanations.

As mentioned in the preceding chapter, many complex medical words are self-explanatory—if you know a little Greek or Latin, which almost all medical professionals do by virtue of having learned medical terminology. Even a rudimentary understanding of a word's origin can be useful in explaining the word to others, especially if a three-stage explanation is used. Take the word "*leukocyte.*"

1. What it is*:* A leukocyte is a white blood cell.

Derivation: *"Leukocyte" comes from the Greek root meaning "white, or light, bright, brilliant and clear." (The apostle Luke, patron saint of physicians, got his name from the same Greek root.) (Haubrich 2003)*

2. What it does: *White blood cells help to defend the body against harmful bacteria and other bad cells in the blood.*

3. How it does it: *They do it by trapping or engulfing them.*

Analogy: They're like the neighborhood police.

The stories behind words are never ending. Learning a few of the Greek and Latin derivations of words common to your practice is one more tool for mastering the art of the explanation. (But don't overdo it, or you'll come across as pedantic.)

Here are a few other nuggets of medical terminology, taken from *Medical Etymology,* by O. H. Perry Pepper, MD (Pepper 1949) and from William S. Haubrich (Haubrich 2003).

Caesarean: *an eponym, using the name Caesar, for a surgical method of delivery . . . based on the claim that Julius Caesar was thus brought into the world.*

Deltoid: *applied to the deltoid muscle because of its triangular shape (Greek letter of triangular shape). The delta of a river is so named for the same reason.*

Solar plexus: *comes from sol, meaning sun; and plexus, or something woven. In this instance the nerves are supposed to radiate like the rays of the sun. (Haubrich 2003)*

25. Avoid distasteful comparisons.

After learning he had advanced cancer, the bicyclist Lance Armstrong was told by his oncologist, "I'm going to kill you. Every day, I'm going to kill you, and then I'm going to bring you back to life. We're going to hit you with chemo, and then hit you again, and hit you again. You're not going to be able to walk. We're practically going to have to teach you to walk again after we're done." (Reisfield and Wilson 2004)

Okay, this is an extreme example. But warlike analogies are commonplace in medicine. We "marshal forces" to "defeat" this or "combat" that. Words like "attack," "enemy," "weapons," "fight," "battle," "poison," and "kill" permeate our conversations with patients. The general is the health professional, the battlefield is the patient's body, and weapons range from chemical to biological to nuclear.

Analogies, metaphors, and other types of comparisons are not merely convenient tools for intellectually explaining complex ideas. All can be emotionally loaded. They can help to lay the foundation for a person's emotional relationship to a procedure or illness.

For example, when a provider compares the aggressiveness of two cancers to a "poodle or a Rottweiler," the emotional impact upon the person preempts any clarity of understanding. Or likening an angioplasty to a Roto-Rooter procedure is frightening. Mention Roto-Rooter and many people will envision a long coil dragged across a lawn and used to violently bore into a fouled drainpipe. The analogy doesn't do justice to the great delicacy of the heart procedure.

Fortunately, war and other violent metaphors, which have long been a staple of medicine, are giving way to more nuanced and sensitive comparisons. Illness is sometimes compared to an unpredictable journey. Going on a journey is much more apt than going to war. Journeys to the unknown are filled with surprises and revelations, marked by ambiguity and insecurity. All of our fortitude may be needed to complete them. There are detours and setbacks, where moments of fear are offset by moments of great fulfillment. Wars are meant only to be won, and they often aren't. Journeys are meant to be lived and experienced, whatever the final destination.

26. Dispel the myth that to simplify automatically means to dumb down.

Suppose someone asked you to describe the appearance of a cell as seen through a light microscope. Then they asked you to describe the same cell as seen through an electron microscope. The descriptions of what you saw would differ dramatically. But would one be any less accurate than the other?

Not really. They are merely different perspectives. Why, then, do professionals often mistake a "low-power" explanation for dumbing something down?

Partly it's because medical specialists often view the world—at least their area of expertise—through an electron microscope. Every tiny detail *seems* indispensable to accuracy. But most of the world still views medicine through a light microscope, at best. And that is often the best place to start from.

6

TALKING ABOUT RISK

Accurately explaining risk is one of the toughest of all communication challenges. The mathematics inherent in risk analysis is just one of the difficulties.

How you explain it depends in large part on who you're explaining it to. Patients and clients comfortable with the paternalistic tradition of medicine might be more than happy to let you size up the risks and then advise them about what to do. Younger, educated, consumer-minded patients may expect you to lay out the statistics in as unbiased a manner as possible so they can make the best decision for themselves. Some number-savvy patients may want to know more than does the average patient, down to the actual sample size or, in rare cases, *p* values.

The mathematics of computing risk can be complicated— the *perception* of risk even more so. Even medical professionals can be misled by the way risk is communicated. Brochures from pharmaceutical companies, for example, may present risk in a way that is technically accurate but that puts a drug in an artificially favorable light. Stating exactly the same risk differently can dramatically change one's perception of the drug—even to the point of influencing whether a veterinarian or physician prescribes it.

For example, if you were told that a medication for high blood pressure reduced a patient's chance of dying from heart disease within five years by about 20 percent, you might find that pretty impressive. But if you were told instead that the same drug lowered the death rate from heart disease from 7.8 percent to 6.3 percent, it might seem a lot less impressive. Yet the different numbers describe exactly the same mathematical risk. How the likelihood of adverse side effects from such drugs is presented is important too.

Although communicating risk to laypeople has been extensively researched, studies on the topic point to no clear consensus on the best way to present risk in most cases. Nevertheless, a few general do's and don'ts seem to hold true for most situations.

27. Use absolute rather than relative risk estimates.

As the example above—the drug for high blood pressure—shows, the problem is not so much that statistics can lie but that the same ones can be employed to tell the "truth" in different ways, each with the potential to differently influence a patient's decision.

On one hand, the drug reduced a patient's chance of dying from heart disease within five years by about 20 percent.

On the other hand, the drug lowered the actual death rate within five years from 7.8 percent to 6.3 percent.

Both figures describe exactly the same mathematical risk. The first (about a 20 percent reduction) is called "relative" risk. It is the *percentage* decrease between the two groups—6.3 and 7.8. That is 19.2 percent. (We're calling this "about 20 percent.")

This is calculated by taking the difference between the two numbers (1.5) and dividing it by 7.8:
$(7.8 - 6.3) / 7.8 = .192$

The drug *seems* to be highly beneficial, indeed! The problem is that relative risk tells you nothing about real risk. The actual difference between the groups, as we saw in calculating the relative risk, is 1.5 percent. This number paints a much less rosy picture of the drug's effectiveness. Only 1.5 percent more of the drug-takers lived for five years than did those not taking the drug.

Even articles in peer-reviewed journals may stack the statistical deck and report only relative risk, thereby making the results of trials seem more impressive than they actually are. The accurate reporting of results is also clouded by the fact that many drug articles are ghostwritten by people paid by the pharmaceutical companies.

Several years ago, a group of researchers examined about 350 randomized clinical trials of new treatments reported in five major medical journals. Only 18 of the papers considered absolute risk reduction.

One of the researchers concluded, "The public expects advertisers to use the most flattering statistics to bolster claims of effectiveness in promoting products. However, most of us expect that medical journals will provide complete reporting of all important aspects of research on a new treatment. Without more comparative data, readers may be basing their decisions to use a new treatment on incomplete information." (Mayor 2002)

One example the paper cites is a study that concluded that the risk for blindness in a diabetic patient over five years if treated with conventional therapy was 2 percent. That is, 2 in every 100 patients in the study became blind. However, blindness in a group of diabetics treated with a new intensive therapy was 1 percent. That is, 1 in every 100 patients became blind.

The relative risk is 50 percent. That is, intensive therapy reduces the risk for blindness by half, according to this study.

But the absolute difference is 1 percent. In other words, in absolute terms, intensive therapy reduces the five-year risk for blindness by that much.

The author concluded, "Without any qualification, both statements ('reduced the risk by 1%' and 'reduced the risk by 50%') could be construed as representing either an absolute or relative difference. But most important, note the difference in 'feel.' A statement of 'reduced the risk by 1%' does feel like a smaller effect than 'reduced the risk by 50%.'" (American College of Physicians 2009)

Medical professionals sometimes rely on relative risks simply because these are often cited in pharmaceutical publications. Press releases from the companies also often use relative estimates, which then end up being reported in the media. This sometimes sends people to providers armed with overly optimistic misinformation. It's not easy to explain how facts can be accurate while the conclusions drawn from them are wrong—or at least misleading. Discussing absolute rather than relative risk with patients and clients—and taking time to explain the difference—is one way to begin to address this persistent problem in risk communication. And these considerations apply equally whether you're talking about the risk or safety of a procedure, a drug or other medical decision.

28. Don't use verbal descriptions of risk.

Medical professionals sometimes try to avoid statistics altogether by verbally describing risk. They use phrases like "The chance of side effects is minor" or "There is a significant chance you'll benefit from this procedure." This only complicates the communication because laypeople almost always exaggerate verbal descriptions of risk for the better or for the worse. They often interpret "minimal" to mean never and "significant" to mean always. Try to avoid words and phrases such as "likely," "unlikely," "very common," "it's possible," "possibly," and "in a small number of cases."

DON'T SAY

There are rarely serious side effects from this medication.

The layperson often hears this and thinks, "Whew! There are never any serious side effects from this medication. Sign me up."

DO SAY

For every 1000 people treated with this drug, 4 developed side effects that didn't require medical treatment.

DON'T SAY

The sedative that will be used during the procedure sometimes has side effects.

The layperson often hears this and concludes, "That's the last thing I need on top of already feeling so bad."

DO SAY

For every 5,000 people treated with this drug, 2 developed side effects that required hospitalization.

29. Be careful when using the words "risk" and "chance."

Studies suggest that most people go by the dictionary definition of "risk," or the possibility of something *bad* happening. But in statistics the term applies equally to bad and good outcomes. For example, the "risk of response" to a drug can just as easily refer to a favorable response as to a negative one. But laypeople almost always think it means bad. Either avoid the term or try to pair "risk" with "benefit" so patients can make sense of the potential trade-offs. Similarly, the word "chance" is open to ambiguous interpretation.

Here are a couple of examples of how risk issues can be addressed clearly without use of the word "risk."

Patient: *I'm worried about any side effects of the drug.*

Health professional: *One way to look at it is like this. About two in every hundred people who take it experience some nausea.*

Patient: *Does the procedure carry a lot of risk?*

Health professional: *It has both risks and benefits. For example, about five in every thousand people who undergo the procedure have complications that go away on their own. On the other hand, about one in every thousand people who undergo the procedure develops complications that require hospitalization.*

30. State both the "gain" and the "loss" scenarios—that is, both the upside and the downside of the risks.

When people are told that those undergoing a treatment have a 90 percent chance of survival, most want it. But when the same treatment is described as being associated with a 10 percent chance of death, most don't. Research consistently finds that the use of gain versus loss frames can influence decision making. Therefore, you should use them both. (Fagerlin, Ubel et al. 2007)

31. If you have the choice, use frequencies rather than percentages when talking about risk.

Numerous studies have shown that both clinicians and patients understand risk information better if it is presented as frequencies (5 in 100 people experienced side effects) rather than as percentages (five percent), perhaps because frequencies appear more people-friendly. (Fagerlin, Ubel et al. 2007)

DON'T SAY

Seventy percent of the people who had this type of surgery said it relieved most of their back pain.

DO SAY

Seven in ten people who had this type of surgery said it relieved most of their back pain.

DON'T SAY

About one-half of one percent of those who take the medication develop ringing in the ears.

DO SAY

About one in every two hundred people who take the medication develops ringing in the ears.

32. Use consistent denominators when talking about multiple risks.

If you're talking about only one risk, it doesn't appear to matter whether you say "one in a hundred" or "ten in a thousand." If you find yourself talking to a patient about several different risks in the same conversation, don't say "one in a hundred" for one case and "ninety in a thousand" for the next. Convert both examples to "in a hundred" or "in a thousand."

DON'T SAY

I understand you're not sure whether it's better to continue taking the old drug or to try the new drug. One way to look at it is that six in a hundred people who took the old drug experienced a reduction in symptoms. Nine hundred in a thousand people who took the new formulation experienced a reduction in symptoms.

DO SAY

I understand you're not sure whether it's better to take the old drug or the new drug. One way to look at it is that six in a hundred people who took the old formulation experienced a reduction in symptoms. Nine in a hundred people who took the new formulation experienced a reduction in symptoms.

33. Use time spans if feasible when talking about risks.

The time span over which a risk is computed can greatly affect a person's perception of risk. It's difficult for people to extrapolate risks from one time span to another. (Fagerlin, Ubel et al. 2007)

For example, telling people that they have a 33 percent risk of serious injury during their lifetime if they don't use car seat belts leads to much higher seat belt use than telling them the much smaller risk of serious injury by not wearing seat belts during a single trip. (Fagerlin, Ubel et al. 2007)

Here is a comparative look at poor, better, and best risk communication. (Each description refers to the outcome of a different study.) (Skolbekken 1998; Hollnagel 1999)

Poor Risk Communication

People with high cholesterol can rapidly reduce their risk of having a first time heart attack by 31 percent and their risk of death by 22 per cent by taking a widely prescribed drug. (Skolbekken 1998)

In this instance, the use of relative risk estimates (percentages rather than frequencies) magnifies the benefit of the drug. The word "risk" is embraced rather than avoided, and no time span is given for the duration of the study of the individuals in question.

Better Risk Communication

People with high cholesterol can rapidly reduce their [absolute] risk of having a first time heart attack by 1.9 percent and their [absolute] risk of death by 0.9 percent by taking a widely prescribed drug.

Although much improved by the use of absolute risk reduction, the inclusion of percentages rather than frequencies muddies the meaning for many listeners. The word "risk" is still used, and no time span is given.

Best Risk Communication

"If 100 people like you are given no treatment for 5 years, 92 will live and eight will die. Whether you are one of the 92 or one of the eight, I don't know. Then, if 100 people like you take a certain drug every day for 5 years, 95 will live and five will die. Again, I don't know whether you are one of the 95 or one of the five."

This explanation avoids many of the common pitfalls of risk communication. It states the absolute risks as frequencies rather than percentages, avoids the word "risk," uses a consistent denominator (100), and avoids verbal descriptions of risk. In addition, it acknowledges uncertainty, gives a time span for the risk, and describes the upside and downside of the risk.

34. When talking about risk, don't offer gratuitous assurances such as "There's really nothing to worry about"—unless there really isn't. If there are known safety issues, acknowledge them.

When it comes to risk, health professionals are frequently tempted to speak in terms of certainty because that's what the public expects from them. But catering to this temptation only perpetuates the myth that science is built on certainty rather than probability. To make a statement without mentioning uncertainty is close to saying it *is* certain.

For decades, officials and experts have assumed it is their job to reassure the public about risk. Whether the risk is that of certain drugs, bird flu, or mad cow disease, this history of "not to worry" is a history of false assurances. It has left a deep mistrust in its wake. When people are facing real danger, don't tell them not to worry. As risk communication expert Peter Sandman advises, don't enable their denial—or your own. Acknowledge uncertainty, share dilemmas—the dilemmas that you as an expert face—and offer people ways to feel that they are part of the solution.

DON'T SAY

I can say completely honestly that I shall go on eating beef and my children will go on eating beef because there is no need to be worried. (Statement made in May 1990 by John Gummer, British agriculture minister, during an interview about mad cow disease aired on BBC-TV.)

What he might have wished he'd said

There is still a lot we don't know about mad cow disease. Although public health scientists are looking into the possible connection between infected cows and human disease, evidence thus far has not shown a connection.

DON'T SAY

The current outbreak is no reason to alter your diet. Your chance of contracting E. coli food poisoning is less than your chance of getting hit by lightning.

DO SAY

Although the food supply is generally safe, this outbreak reminds us of the need to take precautions whenever we prepare poultry or other meat.

DON'T SAY

A new study to the contrary, the vast amount of evidence suggests that this drug is very safe. There's no good reason to stop taking it.

DO SAY

On the basis of this study alone, those benefiting from the drug should not stop taking it but should call their doctor immediately if they experience stomach pain, dizziness, or trouble breathing.

35. Although professionals may think in terms of rational, or mathematical, risk, many laypeople follow their instincts. That doesn't mean their fears are "irrational."

After landing at Newark Liberty International Airport, Continental Airlines flight attendants used to announce something like, "The safest part of your travel day is now over. Please be careful driving home." Every time, heads would whip around and passengers would stare at each other quizzically, as if to ask, "What is she talking about?"

For people who fear flying but love to drive, it's no use telling them that travel by air is actually thousands of times safer, because that's not how it *feels*. Let's face it: feelings, — "instinctual fear," for example—helped our species survive for tens of thousands of years. So our feelings are pretty deeply rooted. Statistics, on the other hand, were invented yesterday. It takes a brave soul to defy instincts and put his or her faith in abstract numbers.

The point is, it is often unfair—not to mention unproductive—to dismiss another's instinctual fear as irrational.

If you find yourself met by parents skeptical of vaccines, for example, do yourself and them a favor by not dismissing them as irrational. Nothing is irrational, in principle, about fearing a foreign substance being injected into one's blood. (There is a long history of public opposition to vaccines, probably for just that reason.) There are some effective ways of addressing this issue.

36. Much fear among the public stems from stories in the media. Don't try to dispel an "anecdotal" fear with statistics. Tell a different story.

Studies show that public perception of risk can be heightened, if not created, by media reports. Rarely are these fears the result of accurately reported statistics. Rather, they are usually based upon stories or anecdotes that may or may not be accurate. The anecdotal story of a child becoming severely ill soon after receiving a vaccination can create an "anecdotal fear" of vaccines—a fear far beyond anything that statistics alone could have done.

Yet medical professionals often throw statistics at "anecdotal" risks. Like instinctual fears, anecdotal fears are often immune to numbers.

But countervailing anecdotes can go a long way toward influencing a layperson's perception of risk.

Increasingly, scientists seem to be using this strategy in talking about vaccines. Rather than using statistics to try to refute anecdotal stories of children seemingly harmed by vaccines, many scientists are using the opposing narrative: describing the outbreaks of preventable disease among children who were not vaccinated.

Statistics madden many laypeople in part because probability is, by nature, a measure of uncertainty, which is just the opposite of what people expect. The dilemma is summed up in the following newspaper headline: "Mayor says poor forecasting doomed city; weather service says it gave its best effort." The mayor had apparently mistaken a prediction for certainty.

While professionals often lament the public's demand for absolute certainty, experts have historically made the problem worse by downplaying the uncertainty of scientific conclusions. By doing so, they not only mislead the public but also invite skeptics to manipulate the public by exploiting inherent uncertainties of the scientific method.

Political consultant Frank Luntz once advised his clients, "Should the public come to believe that the scientific issues are settled, their views about global warming will change accordingly. Therefore, you need to continue to make the lack of scientific certainty a primary issue in the debate . . . The scientific debate is closing [against us] but not yet closed."

If doctors, economists, engineers, and other professionals better explained the role of uncertainty in science, more of the public would recognize it for the strength that it is rather than the weakness that dogs explanations of risk.

37. Take time to explain the difference between association and causation whenever the issue arises.

A recent study linked obesity in children to television viewing. Many people concluded that watching too much television caused the children to become obese. Few newspaper articles raised the possibility that already obese children may have tended to gravitate toward television, perhaps because they weren't fond of running around or playing outside.

Here are a couple of classic examples illustrating the fallacy of confusing cause with association, with a touch of humor to boot.

In certain beach communities, ice cream sales and shark attacks increase at the same time of year. Does that mean that (a) the shark attacks cause ice cream sales to increase? Or (b) does selling people more ice cream make sharks attack, or (c) none of the above? (Obviously, sharks have taken over the ice cream business!)

There is evidence that the number of dental cavities among elementary school children increases along with their vocabulary size. Does this mean that one causes the other? (Another obvious one—clearly, dentists are the secret suppliers of increased vocabularies.)

7

THE VIRTUES OF SILENCE

If you want to be heard, stop talking. Believe it or not, your silence can even be more powerful than your words.

Studies have shown that, more than any other part of the interaction, good listening skills on the part of health care professionals leave clients and patients with the greatest satisfaction. More specifically, studies indicate that patients and clients are most positive about those encounters in which practitioners adhere to the three guidelines that follow. (Gerteis 1993)

38. Pause before you respond.

When you're talking with someone, pauses can show that you are taking in the speaker's words—especially when you are! Pausing acknowledges that the other person has something important to say that merits careful attention—and deserves a thoughtful, rather than reflexive, reply.

In theory, ten three-second pauses during a conversation of, say, ten minutes, will add only thirty seconds. In practice, showing patients and clients that you have heard them will lessen their need to repeat themselves. (People repeat things when they feel they haven't been heard.) With less need to repeat, the conversation may end up shorter, or at least may become more productive.

Honor especially occasional lengthy, even awkward, pauses. The most revelatory statements often occur after long pauses. Of course, sometimes a client is genuinely stuck and can use an assist, but rushing to the rescue may reflect more your own desire to save yourself from discomfort.

39. Don't formulate a response while the other person is talking.

We often talk to hear ourselves rather than to reach others—or, as has been said, we "deliver monologues in the presence of witnesses." And when we're not talking during a conversation, we're often busy formulating an answer to what another is saying. When we take advantage of both sides of the conversation, we're not really listening. In and out of clinical settings, such behavior is usually counterproductive. Practice conversational generosity.

Sometimes we think we're listening when we're not. If you know exactly what to say the second the other person stops talking, you probably haven't listened very well. It's okay to have to search for the right words when you turn comes. It doesn't mean you're inarticulate. There can be an authenticity born of listening well—that is, the struggle that comes from immersing oneself in the meanings of another's words rather than superficially responding to them. This is especially true in a medical setting, where the meanings of words are often rich, complex, and elusive.

40. Using some of the client's words and phrases shows that you've been listening.

Another way to show people you've heard them is to use some of their own language in responding, even if it's not what you would normally use. (A slightly different take on this recommendation was discussed in Chapter 1.) If pausing is the footing for a conversational bridge between you and another, using borrowed words and phrases are timbers for building it.

41. Know the difference between a good interruption and a bad one.

A third way to increase what clients and patients get from an encounter, studies show, is to interrupt at appropriate points for clarification. It's about the only time people actually like to be interrupted. In contrast, unappreciated interruptions are when you cut a person off in order to say something yourself—as opposed to asking for clarification from them.

These, plus a number of finer behaviors and nuances, can get a conversation off on the right foot. When good listening skills are combined with some of the earlier recommendations about rapport and power, we begin to transform the way we communicate. We will notice the improvement. So will our listeners.

42. If you must interrupt, try using body language before words.

If you must interrupt, first try using body language. It can be just as effective but far less offensive than interrupting verbally. Often, all it takes is a facial expression or a hand gesture (a gently raised finger or an outstretched palm) as if to say, "Wait a second," or stepping forward or otherwise signaling it's your turn to talk. Nonverbal signals allow someone to at least finish his or her thought. The speaker does not feel cut off.

43. If you have to redirect the topic of a conversation, use "transitioning."

Recall the earlier conversation:

Patient: *No, sir, I've never had a heart attack. Supposedly, I worked very hard when I was a young man, young boy. I was doing a man's labor, and I was always told I had a good strong heart and lungs. But the lungs couldn't withstand all the cigarettes*

. . . asbestos and pollution and secondhand smoke and all these other things, I guess.

Physician: *Do you have glaucoma?* (Morse, Edwardsen et al. 2008)

The worst way to change the subject is by ignoring what someone has said and starting a new topic. This totally resets the conversation—like a computer crashing and rebooting itself. It is time-consuming for everyone and annoying to the interrupted party. Instead of completely shutting down one conversation and starting a new one, try to master transitioning.

Transitioning can take practice, but when used correctly, it's beautiful. A transitioning phrase usually picks up on something the speaker has said and turns it in a fresh direction rather than dead-ending the current line of conversation and starting anew. For example, if a patient or client is rambling on about his or her medication, pick up on a salient point and follow it with a question.

DON'T SAY
Wait a minute. Did the medication help?

DO SAY
So you took the medication for five days . . . did you feel any better after that?

DON'T SAY

I understand that, but did physical therapy relieve the pain?

DO SAY

So do you think the physical therapy you're talking about lessened the pain?

44. While listening, relax your muscles of articulation.

Watch any two people in conversation (the Dalai Lama aside) and you will invariably see tensing movements of the listener's jaw muscles. These blazingly fast inflections of facial musculature are a language in themselves, broadcasting all sorts of information about attitude and intent.

The point is that good listening means more than not talking or not interrupting the other person. Hearing requires resting—truly relaxing—your muscles of speech long enough to give your hearing "muscles" priority. This facial language, in turn, transmits a powerful message to the other party: I am not only listening; I am hearing.

Professional speakers often do exercises to warm up their muscles of articulation. This can have a significant effect on the quality of their delivery. Warm-up exercises for listening may be just as important.

Among the few times we tend to focus on hearing are when listening to our favorite radio station, a favorite piece of music, or calming natural sounds, such as a stream or a tropical breeze moving through palm trees. Because this type of listening doesn't require us to respond, we are free to take in sounds deeply in ways we rarely do during conversation.

With practice, we can cultivate a physiology of good listening. We can fine-tune our listening apparatus. When we do, and apply it in conversation, those we speak with will feel truly heard.

45. Take turns asking questions.

As we've seen from many examples in preceding chapters, health-care providers ask the overwhelming majority of primary questions when speaking with patients and clients. The client's or patient's questions, by contrast, are usually follow-ups to the provider's primary questions.

Developing a more symmetrical conversation doesn't mean that the patient and provider need to have equal time—only a sense of equal power and standing. Many studies show that by dominating conversations through interruptions and a preponderance of questions, medical professionals promulgate a highly medical perspective, often at the expense of the patient's own predominantly nonmedical experience and understanding.

Laypeople often cede (without intending to) "speaking rights" during conversations with professionals—that is, they often cede to professionals the power to determine when each party speaks and for how long. Professionals sometimes unconsciously promote asymmetry through interruptions, structured questioning, and other means.

For the professional, the best antidote to this is probably a simple awareness of the big home-field advantage that medical professionals have when talking to laypeople. Once aware of this, most are willing to try to level the playing field by asking more indirect questions, going with the patient's or client's agenda when it's appropriate to do so, and interrupting only in exceptional circumstances.

46. Use the pause to buffer defensiveness.

Occasionally, medical professionals may find themselves on the defensive during a conversation. For that matter, the client or patient may be on the defensive. But increasingly, it seems, professionals find themselves being questioned by laypeople armed with medical information from an increasing number of sources—reliable or not. The combination of more information and less time with medical providers presents a dilemma for both patient and provider. Understandably, frequent challenges by laypeople can occasionally put us on the defensive.

Defensiveness means deflecting, or defending oneself against, what another is saying. We get defensive when we hear things that make us uncomfortable.

In the face of such discomfort, we have two choices: cut the other person off (usually the wrong thing to do) or grin and bear it (usually the right thing to do). As you decide what to do, consider that you will get over the momentary discomfort caused by another's words, but the other party may never get over being brusquely cut off.

As an adrenaline-mediated reaction, defensiveness is difficult to control. Here, the all-purpose pause once again comes in handy. Pauses tend to be a natural buffer against defensiveness, perhaps because they take the edge off the adrenaline rush.

There is a Buddhist teaching about the importance of trying to breathe in deeply rather than deflect what troubles you. When we imagine breathing in the troubling words of another, for example, something strange can happen: we are transformed from a judgmental observer of the conversation to a more compassionate participant. It is as if the warm breath of our inhalation melts defensiveness. It's not a panacea for all defensiveness, but it can be profoundly helpful.

47. Use the "act as if" principle.

What if we find ourselves in a situation where we just can't listen well to what someone is saying? Either we're too tired or, truth be told, we just don't care about what they're saying. We've all been there more often than we'd like to admit.

If all else fails, then just "act as if." Acting as if you're there is perhaps the next best thing to actually being there. And the principle is not all about practicing deceit. There is a psychological method to the "act as if" principle. That is, playing a particular role—a good listener, for example—can actually coax us into that state of mind. We think or pretend ourselves into the role we wish to occupy.

At the very least, use body language that suggests you care. Lean forward, nod your head, make eye contact, and let your face register some emotional response to what the person is saying. Listening this way may not make you hear, but it will at least be welcoming to the speaker. But the real power of the "act as if" principle is that by acting as if we're curious and we care, we open our hearts and minds to the possibility of both.

What's more, "acting as if" can be far more rejuvenating at the end of a long day than showing what we actually feel. Pretending to listen well has a way of inspiring us to do so.

8

COMMUNICATION AND THE ART OF STORY

No matter what your walk of life, storytelling almost always has a place in good communication. Yet over the past century the art of storytelling, long part of the social fabric of many cultures, seems to have waned, especially in industrialized nations such as the United States. Some observers have attributed the decline to the rise in science and technology, which values data and hard information above traditional storytelling narrative and values the exchange of information above the art of conversation. When it comes to information, has the need for speed doomed the art of storytelling? One social commentator wrote, "It is as if something that seemed inalienable to us, the securest among our possessions, were taken from us: the ability to exchange experiences." (Benjamin 1968)

This ability to convey one's experience—storytelling—is, after all, the essence of conversation. In contrast to data dumping, or the positing of facts, authentic storytelling draws much on personal experience and emotion.

Storytelling and conversation depend upon people seeing at least something of themselves in everyone else. In other words, they require that people "relate" to one another. (Tannen 2005) Exposition and the conveying of numbers and data have no such requisite. Imagine the difference, for example, between a bank teller giving your account balances and the same teller "off duty" sharing an impromptu story about her daughter's birthday party.

"A perfectly tuned conversation is like an artistic experience," one observer wrote. "The satisfactions of shared rhythm, shared appreciation of nuance, and the mutual understanding that surpasses the meaning of words exchanged . . . go beyond the pleasure of having one's message understood. A perfectly tuned conversation is a ratification of one's way of being human and proof of connection to other people." (Tannen 2005)

It is perceived lack of human connection in the exchange of data and hard information that can leave patients and clients with a sense that something vital is missing when it comes to communication in a hospital or medical setting. A part of them wants the familiar and comforting connectedness that only storytelling and authentic conversation can offer. They want it especially when talking about illness.

Dana Jennings, an editor for the *New York Times* who wrote of his experiences with prostate cancer, expressed the need for storytelling when he wrote that illness is a "crucible in which we patients are somehow, we hope, reborn.

It's a rite of passage as resonant as any other—a graduation, a baptism, a wedding—and should be treated that way . . . I don't want to hear about another stat, another study." He was tired of having providers "translat[ing] me into an abstraction, to deny my damaged and tiresome flesh-and-bloodness."

But as health professionals are forced to do more in less time, can the "slow knowledge" of storytelling find a secure place? Just as hard data is responsible for much of the success of modern medicine, electronic record keeping can greatly facilitate the exchange of information. As we move toward delivering more information faster, what will become of conversation, storytelling, and the exchange of experiences, all of which are vital to building human relationships? Time will tell.

But as time decides, there are steps that medical professionals can take to nurture conversation in everyday encounters with patients, clients, and others—and, in nurturing conversation, to strengthen the human bonds that are an essential part of healing.

In literary theory as in real life, stories consist of characters, a dilemma, and a "plot" in which some resolution of the dilemma—the "rub"—is sought. Professionals can put this elemental knowledge to work in every conversation by embracing their role in the story of illness.

The good news is that the critical importance of narrative communication—storytelling—is slowly being rediscovered. A recent article in the *Harvard Business Review* praised storytelling as "one of the world's most powerful tools for achieving astonishing results." (Guber 2007) And the notion of narrative medicine is alive and well in many medical schools. But what about in ordinary conversation?

Touted in the press and by corporate visionaries, storytelling is now being lauded by organizational psychologists for its primal power to mobilize and empower listeners. If data informs, story motivates. Good conversation melds the two.

But how is this achieved?

48. Think of yourself as a character in your patient's or client's story, bound by a common dilemma that you are seeking to resolve together.

Although we medical professionals may see ourselves as, first and foremost, objective sources of facts and analysis, we are also de facto characters in our patients' and clients' narratives. We have an appointed role in an unfolding plot of their illness or health. We are as much a part of the patients' stories as they are a part of the stories of our lives. We may be minor or major characters, depending upon the narrative, but we are almost always there. So why not acknowledge it?

Even the simplest of statements during a conversation can reflect our involvement in another's narrative or story.

For example, "Your red blood cell count is low" is a statement of fact, a transmission of information from a presumably neutral source. But the statement "You came to see me because you were feeling unusually tired, we took a blood test, and it showed your red cell count was low" suddenly is peopled with characters—the patient and provider. The statement binds them together in a common story. By doing so, it also lays the groundwork for a conversation instead of a data exchange devoid of context.

49. Acknowledge the "rub" in which you and your patient or client are involved.

Assuming your role as a character in the patient's or client's story is just the first step toward creating a conversation that connects rather than a mere exchange that doesn't. The next step is to acknowledge that you, as a character in this story, are also part of the deepest workings of the narrative.

We learned in elementary school that stories have plots and that plots revolve around the conflict, or rub, to be resolved. As it turns out, most conversations have "plots" and "rubs," too. Nowhere is this truer than in conversations about illness. Why, then, do exchanges so often miss these essential elements of conversation?

For example, the sentence "I'd like to do an X-ray" is the statement of a plan. Compare this with the following:

You've been coughing a lot and have had some chest pain. I would like to run a few tests to get to the bottom of this.

Both the characters and the rub are named. By naming the conflict, we signal our listeners of our involvement. By naming their concern, we also let them know we care.

50. Recognize how you and your patient or client are bound together in a narrative by a shared "plot."

While characters and the conflict are essential to just about every narrative, there is a third ingredient. This is the series of events revolving around the characters' efforts to resolve the story's conflict—the plot. This element, too, is often a part of conversation, for many conversations are simply a continuous form of storytelling. Even a basic if-then statement can suggest plot in a way that simple recital of the facts rarely does. For example, the statement "Take this medication twice a day" has no plot. It is simply a command. But the phrasing "If you take this medication twice a day, there is a much better chance that you will feel better" has a character (the patient) and an if-then plot.

And adding the practitioner can further transform the narrative:

I know you've been feeling a lot of pain lately. If you take this medication two times a day, there is a chance you'll feel much better.

Instead of instructing someone what to do, you have joined their personal narrative. You have become a storyteller.

As these examples indicate, by carefully constructing your sentences, you can join your listeners' stories rather than merely observe them. You have identified with your listeners; you have made a connection. That's what stories do. They join and connect. You have not only joined them in their story; you have helped to tell their story. And nothing is more powerful than when a health-care provider tells the story of his or her client or patient.

SOURCES

Ainsworth-Vaughn, N. (1998). Claiming power in doctor-patient talk. New York, Oxford University Press.

American College of Physicians (2009). "Primer on absolute vs. Relative Differences." Effective Clinical Practice. 2(6).

Aronson, S. M. (2005). "The many words of diabetes mellitus." Medicine and Health Rhode Island.

Banay, G. L. (1948). "An introduction to medical terminology 1. Greek and Latin Derivations." Bull Med Libr Assoc. 36(1): 1-27.

Beck, R. S., R. Daughtridge, et al. (2002). "Physician-patient communication in the primary care office: a systematic review." J Am Board Fam Pract 15(1): 25-38.

Benjamin, W. (1968). Illuminations. New York, Harcourt.

Brunetti, L., J. P. Santell, et al. (2007). "The impact of abbreviations on patient safety." Jt Comm J Qual Patient Saf 33(9): 576-583.

Conklin, M. G. (1912). Conversation: what to say and how to say it. New York and London, Funk & Wagnalls Company.

Fagerlin, A., P. A. Ubel, et al. (2007). "Making numbers matter: present and future research in risk communication." American J Health Behav 31(Supple 1): S47-S56.

Frieden, I. J. and J. C. Dolev (2005). "Medical analogies: Their role in teaching dermatology to medical professionals and patients." Journal of the American Academy of Dermatology 53(5): 863-866.

Gerteis, M. (1993). Through the patient's eyes: understanding and promoting patient-centered care. San Francisco, Jossey-Bass.

Guber, P. (2007). The four truths of the storyteller. Harvard Business Review.

Haubrich, W. S. (2003). Medical meanings: a glossary of word origins. Philadelphia, American College of Physicians.

Hollnagel, H. (1999). "Explaining risk factors to patients during a general practice consultation: Conveying group-based epidemiological knowledge to individual patients." Scandinavian Journal of Primary Health Care 17(1): 3-5.

Johnson, P. and T. S. Johnson (2009). "Improved communications reduce litigation." AAOS Now 3(2).

Lakoff, R. T. (1990). Talking power: the politics of language in our lives. New York, Basic Books.

Mayor, S. (2002). "Researchers claim clinical trials are reported with misleading statistics." British Medical Journal 324(7350): 1353.

Moore, P. J., N. E. Adler, et al. (2000). "Medical malpractice: the effect of doctor-patient relations on medical patient perceptions and malpractice intentions." Western Journal of Medicine 173(October): 244-250.

Morris, G. H. and R. J. Chenail (1995). The talk of the clinic: explorations in the analysis of medical and therapeutic discourse. Hillsdale, N.J., Erlbaum.

Morse, D. S., E. A. Edwardsen, et al. (2008). "Missed opportunities for interval empathy in lung cancer communication." Arch Intern Med 168(17).

Pepper, O. H. P. (1949). Medical etymology: the history and derivation of medical terms for students of medicine, dentistry, and nursing. Philadelphia,, W.B. Saunders Co.

Rao, J. K., L. A. Anderson, et al. (2007). "Communication interventions make a difference in conversations between physicians and patients: a systematic review of the evidence." Medical Care 45(4): 340-349.

Reisfield, G. M. and G. R. Wilson (2004). "Use of Metaphor in the Discourse on Cancer." J Clin Oncol 22(19): 4024-4027.

Rose, S. P. (2003). "How to (or not to) communicate science." Biochem Soc Trans 31(2): 307-312.

Roter, D. and J. A. Hall (2006). Doctors talking with patients/patients talking with doctors: improving communication in medical visits. Westport, Conn., Praeger.

Samora, J., L. Saunders, et al. (1961). "Medical vocabulary knowledge among hospital patients." Journal of Health and Human Behavior 2(summer): 83-92.

Shortland, M. and J. Gregory (1991). Communicating science: a handbook. New York, Wiley.

Skolbekken, J. A. (1998). "Communicating the risk reduction achieved by cholesterol reducing drugs." BMJ 316(7149): 1956-1958.

Tannen, D. (2005). Conversational style: analyzing talk among friends. New York, Oxford University Press.

West, C. (1984). Routine complications: troubles with talk between doctors and patients. Bloomington, Indiana University Press.

Young, M. E., G. R. Norman, et al. (2008). "The Role of Medical Language in Changing Public Perceptions of Illness." PLoS ONE 3(12): e3875.